Praise for *Meditation*

"In *Meditation as Medicine,* Dr. Dharma Singh Khalsa shows us how the tremendous power of medical meditation can heal not only the body but also the mind and soul. I strongly recommend it."

—Deepak Chopra, M.D., author of *How to Know God*

"*Meditation as Medicine* explores one of the most ancient methods of healing known to humankind, whose benefits have been affirmed by hundreds of careful scientific studies. Dr. Dharma Singh Khalsa is a respected physician who skillfully guides us in a journey to greater health. Whether you are a beginner in meditation or a veteran, you will benefit from this very wise book."

—Larry Dossey, M.D., author of
Reinventing Medicine and *Healing Words*

"*Meditation as Medicine* is a new concept, but the techniques that it uses are ancient, part of the wisdom tradition of India. The authors of this book explain those techniques in a clear and engaging manner, making their relevance to the prevention and treatment of disease very obvious. I found much practical advice here."

—Andrew Weil, M.D., author of
Spontaneous Healing and *Eating Well for Optimum Health*

"*Meditation as Medicine* is an extraordinary guide to tapping into the innate healing powers we all have. I highly recommend it to everyone at all levels."

—Judith Orloff, M.D., author of
Dr. Judith Orloff's Guide to Intuitive Healing

"*Meditation as Medicine* is required reading for anyone truly interested in the role of meditation in the healing process."

—Arielle Ford, author of *Hot Chocolate for the Mystical Soul*

"Activate and use your deep natural abilities now with Dr. Khalsa's book *Meditation as Medicine.*"

—Mark Victor Hansen, co-creator, #1 *New York Times* bestselling
Chicken Soup for the Soul series

"Within these very pages is the best knowledge you can find. Everybody must seek it out."

—Yogi Bhajan, Ph.D., master of kundalini and white tantric yoga

Meditation as Medicine

Activate the Power of
Your Natural Healing Force

DHARMA SINGH KHALSA, M.D.

AND

CAMERON STAUTH

FIRESIDE

New York London Toronto Sydney Singapore

Kundalini Research Institute

This Seal of Approval is granted only to those products which have been approved through the KRI Review process for accuracy and integrity of those portions which embody the technology of Kundalini Yoga and 3HO Lifestyle as taught by Yogi Bhajan.

The ideas, procedures, and suggestions in this book are not intended as a substitute for the medical advice of a trained health professional. All matters regarding your health require medical supervision. Consult your physician before adopting the suggestions in this book, as well as about any condition that may require diagnosis or medical attention. The author and publisher disclaim any liability arising directly or indirectly from the use of the book [or of any products mentioned herein].

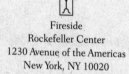

Fireside
Rockefeller Center
1230 Avenue of the Americas
New York, NY 10020

First Fireside Edition 2002

FIRESIDE and colophon are registered trademarks of Simon & Schuster, Inc.

For information regarding special discounts for bulk purchases, please contact Simon & Schuster Special Sales at 1-800-456-6798 or business@simonandschuster.com

Manufactured in the United States of America

1   3   5   7   9   10   8   6   4   2

The Library of Congress has cataloged the Pocket Books edition as follows:
Singh Khalsa, Dharma.
Meditation as medicine: activate the power of your
natural healing force/Dharma Singh Khalsa.
p.   cm.
Includes index.
1. Meditation—Therapeutic use. I. Title.
RC489.M43 S57   2001   615.8'52—dc21   00-68206
ISBN 0-7434-0064-X
0-7434-0065-8 (Pbk)

For my wife, Kirti,
a shining example of love, divinity, and grace.

DHARMA SINGH KHALSA, M.D.

For Gabriel, my magical son,
born the first hour of November 11, 1991.

CAMERON STAUTH

Author's Note

This book is written to help you develop a very high level of physical, mental, emotional, and spiritual health. It can also be used to help you heal from an illness. Of course, it is not a substitute for medical care, but is a very effective adjunct. Many of the patient illustrations in *Meditation as Medicine* are from my clinical work. Other accounts came when I asked the universe to provide me with healing stories. In almost all cases, the person's identity was masked to protect confidentiality.

Dharma Singh Khalsa, M.D.

Contents

Foreword

Joan Borysenko, Ph.D.

Dr. Dharma Singh Khalsa is a brilliant, funny, and gentle physician who has devoted his life to healing through time-tested yogic techniques that are beginning to yield their secrets to medical science. One of my first memories of Dharma is his impromptu performance of Beatles songs at a talent night at a professional conference for which I was the master of ceremonies. Wielding a well-used guitar and wearing his immaculate white turban, he made a wonderful symbol of East meeting West. A childlike joy emanated from him, drawing the audience into a space of delight. The yogic disciplines that Dharma has mastered and practices faithfully have not made him dry and ascetic. Rather, they have allowed him to live life more fully and abundantly, with great mental and physical strength. They can do the same for you.

For almost twenty years I researched the mind/body connection, the pathways through which the mind and emotions affect immunity and other physiological systems. Like many researchers in integrative medicine, my interest in the field stemmed from personal health problems that the best of our powerful modern medicine could not help. Chronic migraine headaches, irritable bowel syndrome, dizziness, anxiety, and an irregular heartbeat made my graduate studies at Harvard Medical School very difficult. Fortunately, my lab partner in physiology was a student of yoga. He suggested that I try some of the same yogic breathing exercises and meditations that Dr. Khalsa outlines so effectively for you. After a few months of practicing these techniques, my symptoms disappeared. I felt more peaceful and joyful than I had believed possible.

My personal experience with meditation and yoga inspired the desire to help others. While an assistant professor at Tufts Medical School in Boston, I taught yoga and meditation to staff, faculty, and students. Then in 1978 I accepted a postdoctoral fellowship at Harvard with Dr. Herbert Benson, with whom I had worked briefly as a graduate student a decade previously. In 1967 I assisted Dr. Benson with his research on biofeedback, in which he demonstrated that blood pressure can be controlled by behavioral means. Then our paths parted. Dr. Benson began to study the physiological effects of meditation, which he called the relaxation response. I studied the pathology of cancer cells, researching ways to make them behave normally.

When my beloved father died of cancer, I realized that I knew a great deal about cancer cells, but almost nothing about the experience of people with cancer and that of their loved ones. Drs. Carl and Stephanie Simonton were just beginning their explorations of mental imagery, attitude, and cancer survival. I joined with Dr. Benson in the hope of contributing something useful to this new field of behavioral medicine and cancer. More than twenty years have passed since that time, and a great deal of medical research on the effects of yoga and meditation has begun to prove their efficacy. While much research remains to be done, you will read of the great strides that have been made in the chapters to follow.

The medical and psychological effects of ancient, time-tested healing techniques from other cultures, including Qi Gong from Chinese medicine and yoga from India, are an area of intense exploration. Dr. Benson's pioneering research on the health benefits of focused attention, which elicit the relaxation response, provided an important first step. Whenever the mind is focused on the here and now, cutting off the anxiety-provoking inner dialogue that conjures images of past troubles or future problems, an integrated hypothalamic response that decreases the fight-or-flight response is initiated. Not only does this response short-circuit needless activation of the stress-producing sympathetic nervous system, it also yields entry into more refined control of the nervous system. For example, the Tibetan practice of *gtumo* yoga enables the meditator to increase body temperature and remain comfortable in freezing temperatures, while essentially naked and wrapped in wet sheets, which soon dry from the body heat generated by gtumo practice. This well-researched physiological effect is a step beyond the relaxation response that serves as a gateway for more sophisticated physiological control.

The next frontier in medical yoga and meditation is outlined by Dr.

Khalsa in these pages. What meditation techniques are especially useful for specific medical conditions? Some research has already been done, but much more remains. Nonetheless, the collected experience of thousands of years suggests that different meditative techniques stimulate specific physical responses. Much of modern medical treatment stems from similar logic. Many accepted treatments are based on demonstrated clinical usefulness, even when the specific physiological mechanisms have yet to be worked out.

In this book, for the first time, a program of Medical Meditation that bridges ancient wisdom with developments in modern science is made available. In the years to come, we will doubtless learn much more about the molecular underpinnings of these practices. Until that time, we can rely on the fact that these time-honored techniques have proved their utility over the thousands of years during which they were developed and practiced.

The practices are clearly outlined and easily learned. The chapter on breathing alone can transform your body and mind. This book is a treasure, presenting techniques that just a few years ago were unavailable to the average person. Use it with confidence. Medical Meditation can help bring about well-being, spiritual healing—a sense of deep connection to life, compassion, and peace of mind—and, in many cases, needed physical healing.

A Personal Prologue

Dharma Singh Khalsa, M.D.

In your hands you hold a book that can change your life. Using meditation as medicine has helped hundreds of thousands of people around the globe recover from illness, resolve emotional conflicts and reach their optimal potential in mind, body and spirit.

My own experience with Medical Meditation, the type presented in this book, goes back to August 1978. After finishing my anesthesiology residency at the University of California, San Francisco, I moved to Albuquerque, New Mexico, for my first hospital position. I recall very clearly asking the wife of a friend where I could find a yoga class. At the time I was a practitioner of basic yoga and the Transcendental Meditation technique. Leslie simply pointed to a listing in a local alternative newspaper and said, "I hear that's a good one." So off I went. Little did I know that this class would totally transform my life. It was a session in kundalini yoga and meditation as taught by Yogi Bhajan. The facilitator of the class that day was a young man with a beard and a turban.

For some reason, I had a sense that this was exactly the right thing to do. Finding your dharma, or true path, I think, depends on having a feel for your own destiny, so that you know it when you see it. One fine day, you just happen to peek through a crack in your world—and there it is.

When I began to do kundalini yoga and meditation—essentially the same form of meditation that I later adapted as Medical Meditation—it changed me forever. I experienced a very elevated state, mentally, physically, and spiritually, which felt very healing to me. This feeling is so indescribable and indefinable that I think it makes the most sense to describe it only in terms that are allegorical or amorphous, such as "highest self."

I'm certain you know what I mean. You've felt it. You may not have felt it for years, maybe not since your childhood, but you still remember it. Once you've felt it, the feeling's there forever.

For about two years, I continued to practice kundalini yoga and meditation almost daily, but had not yet decided to integrate it absolutely into the fabric of my life, personally and professionally. Over this same period of time, I had also become very interested in the religion that is often associated with kundalini yoga, Sikhism. Kundalini yoga and Sikhism are two very different things; they both originated in India, but one is an ancient science, and the other is a religion. In America virtually all Western Sikhs practice kundalini, but the majority of the world's 15 million Sikhs, most of whom live in India, do not practice kundalini. One major reason that many of America's kundalini practitioners have converted to Sikhism is because Sikhism is the religion of Yogi Bhajan, America's only kundalini yoga master, who was raised in the Sikh tradition in India.

Because of the powerful influence of Yogi Bhajan, the Mahan Tantric (or highest living yoga master in the world), if a person practices kundalini in America, he or she is sure to be exposed to Sikhism. Personally, the more I saw of it, the more I liked it. I loved the universality of it, the assumption that there is only one God, but that it can be equally proper to address this God as Allah, or Jehovah, or God, or Vishnu. I also loved the religion's strong and simple moral code: Help other people. In addition, I was captivated by its lack of a punitive, judgmental attitude, and its insistence that being happy is as godly as being holy. I discovered that Sikhism, the world's fifth-largest religion, is short on dogma but full of heart. Still, I wasn't quite ready to take the leap and commit completely to the vigorous and altruistic Sikh lifestyle, including wearing the traditional turban, which helps keep kundalini energy elevated.

Before deciding to adopt Sikhism, I sought the advice of the fabled Yogi Bhajan, whom I'd never met. I'd heard he was a man of ultimate honesty, and that if he thought this wasn't right for me, as an individual, he'd tell me so.

I drove over to a house where he was staying in Albuquerque. What happened next felt very strange, almost surrealistic. He was lying on a couch in the house amid a large group of people. As I entered the room, it seemed as if the Red Sea of people between us parted, and that I glided over to him, not on my own power, in a movement that felt nothing like walking.

But before I could speak, all I could see were his luminous eyes as he said, "Tell me, Doctor, how much *money* do you make?" To this day I'm not sure why he said what he did, but in that brief moment I was blasted out of the conventional doctor-box forever.

Then he closed his eyes and went into a deep meditation, and for some reason I didn't feel at all shut out. In fact, I felt as if he were including me, on a level much deeper than the one on which a host usually includes his guest.

When he opened his eyes, I was waiting for him to say something profound.

He said, "Let's go to the movies."

So we did, along with a number of other people. Then something else unusual happened.

I went to the restroom, and as I was washing my hands, Yogi Bhajan emerged from one of the stalls. He said, "We are together." Then I heard him say, "Again." I started to say, "Yes, again." Stopped. I realized that he hadn't actually *said* "Again"—even though I'd *heard* it just as distinctly as the rest of his statement. Of course, this could have been my imagination, but I'd never before imagined anything at all like this. Did he mean again as in a previous life or again as in today? I was beginning to think that either this was the most intuitive, tuned-in person I'd ever met, or that I was in the Twilight Zone.

Two weeks later, I went to Espanola, New Mexico, the picturesque desert village that is Yogi Bhajan's retreat. For the first time, I donned a turban and the traditional white clothing that Sikhs wear. I wanted to talk to Yogi Bhajan. I was concerned that this striking form of dress would change my identity at the hospital. In addition, if I converted, I would have to change my name to Khalsa, or Pure One, because that's the traditional last name of all Sikhs, who are members of the "Brotherhood of the Khalsa." These would be major changes for me—hard ones.

Even so, they were changes that I hoped would help me find spiritual fulfillment. As I pondered my destiny, or dharma, I couldn't help but think about my father, who had, I feared, died spiritually unfulfilled at the relatively young age of sixty-three from pancreatic cancer. I also thought about my two uncles, men of achievement, but maybe not fulfillment, dead also at sixty-three. Sixty-three didn't seem that far away.

I approached Yogi Bhajan, who noted my turban. He said, "Do you think you can go before the public like that?"

"It may take some time," I said.

"Time," he replied. "What is time? Do you think sixty-three years is a long time?"

I had begun to say no when I realized that he had pulled the number 63 out of thin air, or out of my mind, and I was very startled and amazed. But then my amazement seemed to congeal into a laserlike beam of understanding that traveled straight from my forehead to that of Yogi Bhajan. At that moment, I felt suddenly capable of committing myself to a new life and a new name.

I wrote down my American name, and my date and place of birth, and gave it to Yogi Bhajan. He performed a yogic calculation, wrote my spiritual name, or Sikh name, on a piece of paper, and handed it to me. It said, "Dharma Singh: A pure lion on a victorious path." Another way to interpret it would be: "A man who fights like a lion for his destiny."

At the instant I saw the name, the buzzing, floating feeling in my forehead intensified, and I felt as if I had for the first time in my life opened my "third eye," or sixth chakra—the only part of me that can see without illusion.

Then and there, my life changed forever. I knew that I could take the truths I had learned from advanced Medical Meditation and apply them successfully to the world of modern medicine, and that matters of dress and status were utterly trivial compared to what I hoped to achieve.

No longer would I have to be content with using modern drugs as an anesthesiologist to make patients unconscious. Now I could truly help them become conscious human beings.

I became Dharma.

Throughout these ensuing twenty-plus years I have used Medical Meditation to elevate myself and help my patients heal. Your journey to healing lies within you. In your hands you hold the key to the success of that journey. Using *Medical Meditations* will activate the power of your natural healing force, the force that allows your body, mind, and spirit to heal themselves.

Meditation is a natural physiological event, well studied and actually quite simple to perform. As I will show you in this book, it is also medically specific. The healing energy Medical Meditation generates involves the complete mind-body-spirit connection. It creates a state of exaltation, the essence of which ultimately creates total health and regeneration.

It is your birthright as a human being to be healthy, happy, and whole. Now is the time to claim this power. *Meditation as Medicine* provides all the tools you will ever need. Let us begin.

> *May the long time sun shine upon you,*
> *all love surround you,*
> *and the pure light within you*
> *guide your way on.*

PART ONE

Healing with
Medical Meditation

CHAPTER ONE

Introducing Medical Meditation

Just before dawn, in the intense quiet outside my desert home, slight sun and deep shadow swirl together, coloring the eastern sky a streaked gray, with a slash of brightness at the horizon, promising light. This is not the darkest, but the lightest hour of the night.

As the most distant stars begin to blink off, warmth fights the night-time chill, and the mix of hot and cold twirls in a breeze that touches my face. As the stillness of night gives way, cardinals and finches begin to tentatively test the quiet. In the hills and canyons behind my house, their songs herald the sun. It reminds me of a proverb: "Faith is the bird that feels the light, and sings while the dawn is still dark."

I discovered that if I listened carefully to the birds that lived around my house, and whistled their own cries—not just generic birdcalls, but each bird's own signature song—they would often answer. A cardinal calls; I do my best to mimic his cry, and I am rewarded with a reply: "Whit-chewww! Whit-whit-whit-whit!" As we trade sounds, I focus on the exquisite beauty of the desert that surrounds my rural Tucson, Arizona, home. I see that the rugged perfection of the desert, with its infinite capacity for survival, reflects the most fundamental secrets of healing: balance, regeneration, and the ability to change.

I feel certain that if I can help my patients find these powers in themselves, I can help them heal. And on this day I will need these powers badly, because a patient is coming to me who has lost faith that a new day will always dawn for her. She has a terrible medical problem, and fears, quite realistically, that she will be paralyzed for the rest of her life.

Sadly, the grip that paralysis holds on her has practically stopped her life, even while she still draws breath. She is still struggling through the motions of life, but she doesn't have much heart or hope left. She is clinging desperately to her old habits and perceptions, as if change itself were death.

I look to the horizon, now pink with blue, close my eyes, and ask God to give me the power to speak to this frightened person in her own language, so that I can reach her center and reignite the spark that has been snuffed. In my mind I can see the sun, brilliant and pulsing, still on the other side of the world.

A force begins to flow into me as I begin my first mantra of the day: "Ong Namo, Guru Dev Namo" ("I bow before my highest self"). It's always my first mantra. On this day, I mean this mantra with all my heart, because I know that only my highest self—the part of me that can feel the universal spirit—can help heal my patient's tortured soul and broken body.

As time falls away, I chant, "Ong Namo, Guru Dev Namo." I can speak the words in English, "I bow before my highest consciousness," but it would not have the same physical effect. The ancient Sanskrit words that I chant every morning have a very specific physiological action. The reverberative sounds in them vibrate the pituitary, just above the roof of my mouth, which changes the secretions of this master gland of the endocrine system.

Obviously, the ancient yoga masters who devised this mantra had no anatomic knowledge of the pituitary, but they did know that the Ong Namo mantra worked. Quite simply, it made people feel more like themselves— their true selves, their highest selves. It doesn't concern me that the ancient masters didn't know about the pituitary, because even today doctors don't know why some of their treatments work—they still don't know why aspirin stops pain, they just know that it does.

The ancient yoga masters taught that this mantra and others should be chanted before dawn. They did not know that the hours just before sunrise are critical to the body's balance of hormones and neurotransmitters, which the pituitary influences. Modern neuroscientists know now that these are the hours during which the endocrine and neurotransmitter balance shifts from relative domination by sleep-inducing melatonin to relative domination by serotonin, norepinephrine, and cortisol. If this shift does not occur smoothly, it can have very distressing, and even disastrous, effects. It can diminish the production of stimulating neurochemicals, and leave people groggy and depressed all day. Or it can have the opposite effect, and cause overproduction of the stress hormone cortisol, which can cause agitation, immune dysfunction, memory loss, and premature aging. The ancient yoga masters knew nothing of the endocrine system, but they did know that there was something magical and empowering in the predawn hours, which they called the ambrosial hours.

As the sun slowly begins to bathe my face in radiance, my sense of personal power, serenity, and intuition continue to expand. I keep meditating, and doing exercises of kundalini yoga. These exercises heighten the presence of life energy, or vitality, which the ancient masters called kundalini. The exercises are the physical element of meditation, and are every bit as important as the mental element, since mind and body are inseparable.

I finish by chanting the Mantra of Ecstasy, "Wahe Guru" ("Out of darkness, into light"). Suddenly a hot knot of fear hits my stomach, hard as a fist. How could I possibly help heal this young woman? She has a spinal injury that is, by all conventional medical reckoning, beyond help. She clearly wants me to work a miracle, but no honest doctor can ever presume that capability.

I vowed over the phone to do whatever I could to help her. But ever since she called, I've been uneasy. Afraid to be totally honest. I was afraid I would let her down, and add to her emptiness. But I pushed down the fear and rationalized it. I went back to my work. On a conscious level, the fear went away.

During my meditation, though, my fear has resurfaced. Maybe my meditative mental state, which is analogous to a hypnotic state, has allowed the fear to break out. Or maybe the yoga I was doing released emotions that I stored in neuropeptides in my abdominal area. I know it may sound like sci-fi to say that emotions can literally be stored in the gut, but the latest neurological research, by Dr. Candace Pert and others, indicates that this astounding mind-body function is quite real. Many of your gut feelings are literally the results of the neurochemicals that abound in your upper intestine.

As quickly as my fear hit, it evaporated. I felt much better, as I always do when meditation lets me release fear or anger. Some people think that meditation is nothing but sitting around feeling blissful, like a latter-day Buddha with a big enlightened smile. But it's not like that. Meditation means opening yourself to the truth. And sometimes the truth hurts.

After I faced my fear, I found myself focusing on my patient in a much clearer, sharper way. Meditation is excellent at removing the obscuring screens of your own personal concerns, and letting you see things the way they really are.

What I see now is a young woman who is suffering more than most people can bear, and who would be grateful for any help she could get. If I can just give to her—give anything—and stop worrying about how much I can give, perhaps I can help her heal.

I open my eyes and feel a rush of compassion for my patient, warm as a wave in the Caribbean. The compassion does not feel like sadness. It feels like joy.

I stand up, and hear the beauty of birds in full concert. The desert, yellow now and vibrating with sun, is alive with the new energy of heat. My day has begun. I am ready. I have gone out of the darkness, into the light.

The Ancient Science and the New Application

When my teacher, Yogi Bhajan, the only master of white tantric yoga in the world, was a boy in India, his yoga master told him to climb into a tree. At that time, it was his teacher who was the only living master, or Mahan Tantric, of white tantric yoga, which is the ultimate yoga to purify and uplift one's being. Therefore Yogi Bhajan, who was then known merely as Harbhajan Singh, dutifully climbed the tree. His master left—and remained gone for three days and three nights. When the master finally returned, his dedicated student was still in the tree. The master asked the student what he had learned. The boy replied that he had learned how to collect water from the rain showers, and which branches the monkeys liked to sleep on. His master nodded, and spoke no more of the experience. But the master continued to teach the boy the secrets of advanced meditation, which had been taught to him—in utmost secrecy—by the yoga masters of the prior era.

For this continued teaching, Yogi Bhajan was profoundly grateful. He felt he was paying a small price for this important knowledge, which had been personally passed from master to student for centuries, and zealously guarded.

The secrets of advanced meditation were shrouded in secrecy because of respect for, and even fear of, their innate power. Just as governments guard state secrets of power, the ancient yoga masters guarded these secrets of spiritual power. They believed that power has the capacity to corrupt, and that it would be disastrous for the wrong person to learn these secrets.

Therefore, these advanced meditations were hidden from the common man, and made available only to disciples proven to have pure hearts. Proving one's purity, of course, required great discipline. For example, as young Yogi Bhajan, or Harbhajan Singh, rose in worldly status—as a prominent athlete, government official, and military officer—he was continually tested by those who guarded the secrets of advanced meditation. Once, when Harbhajan Singh was a high-ranking military officer—and already a renowned yogi—he sought to learn a particular set of meditations, or *kriya,* from an erudite teacher. He called on the teacher for months, but was never given an audience. Finally, the teacher sent a message that Harbhajan Singh should personally make him a carrot pudding, and deliver it to him, five miles on foot, barefoot, every day for one week. Each day the respected officer left his car and driver five miles from the teacher, took off his boots, and walked the dusty, hot path in his starched uniform, carrying the pudding. At last, he was granted the knowledge.

After many more years of practice and service, Yogi Bhajan was recognized as the Mahan Tantric, the world's leading authority on yoga and meditation. As such, he became the most recent member of the golden chain— the lineage of yoga masters, just one every generation, who have carried forward the practice of advanced meditation.

Then, in 1969, Yogi Bhajan undertook a revolutionary act. Having moved to America, he broke with tradition and began to teach the secrets of Medical Meditation to anyone who had a sincere interest. He offered a simple explanation for breaking the code of silence: "We are in the desert, and I have some water."

Since that time, partly as a result of Yogi Bhajan's efforts, the American interest in meditation has grown geometrically. Currently, over 50 million Americans, or 19 percent of the population, engage in meditation.

Until very recently, most of the interest in meditation has been focused on the most basic, fundamental forms of meditation: Transcendental Meditation, popularized by the Beatles, and the relaxation response, popularized by Harvard's Dr. Herbert Benson. Dr. Benson, who directed a postgraduate course I took at Harvard Medical School, was chiefly concerned with isolating the most obvious healing aspect of meditation, and therefore focused his research almost solely upon simple, worry-free relaxation. In so doing, he made meditation palatable to the medical community. Due to Dr. Benson's work over the past twenty-five or thirty years, a large body of studies has indicated clearly that basic meditation, including the relaxation response, is an extremely viable treatment approach. Hundreds of studies have been performed, and they indicate the following:

- Meditation creates a unique hypometabolic state, in which the metabolism is in an even deeper state of rest than during sleep. During sleep, oxygen consumption drops by 8 percent, but during meditation, it drops by 10 to 20 percent.
- Meditation is the only activity that reduces blood lactate, a marker of stress and anxiety.
- The calming hormones melatonin and serotonin are increased by meditation, and the stress hormone cortisol is decreased.
- Meditation has a profound effect upon three key indicators of aging: hearing ability, blood pressure, and vision of close objects.
- Long-term meditators experience 80 percent less heart disease and 50 percent less cancer than nonmeditators.
- Meditators secrete more of the youth-related hormone DHEA as they age than nonmeditators. Meditating forty-five-year-old males have an average of 23 percent more DHEA than nonmeditators, and meditating females have an average of 47 percent more. This helps decrease stress, heighten memory, preserve sexual function, and control weight.
- 75 percent of insomniacs were able to sleep normally when they meditated.
- 34 percent of people with chronic pain significantly reduced medication when they began meditating.

As the body of research on meditation has grown, it's become evident that meditation confers not just strong psychological benefits but also profoundly important physiological benefits. I will go into greater detail on these studies and others in chapter 3.

Another phenomenon that has emerged is that not all meditation is equally effective. For example, most doctors consider techniques such as visualization, guided imagery, progressive relaxation, and affirmations to be forms of meditation, but these techniques lack the medical efficacy of the relaxation response. Similarly, the relaxation response has been shown by studies to be less effective than Transcendental Meditation. A meta-analysis of several hundred studies indicates that Transcendental Meditation exceeds the relaxation response in reducing psychophysical arousal due to stress, decreasing anxiety, increasing mental health, and decreasing drug use. Other studies show that Transcendental Meditation is more effective than the relaxation response at reducing hypertension, reducing mortality in the elderly, and decreasing outpatient visits and medical expenditures.

Similarly, a smaller number of studies indicate that advanced meditation, including Medical Meditation, is more successful than any other form of meditation, including Transcendental Meditation. Some of these studies, though, are ongoing, and have not yet been published. The strongest argument for the superiority of advanced meditation comes from empirical evidence, gleaned from individual clinical practices, such as my own. In my own practice, advanced meditation has clearly outperformed any other form of meditation. When it is used, results are generally more striking, and more immediate.

Due to the progressive nature of my practice, I tend to attract patients who have already participated in other forms of meditation, and these patients are uniformly impressed with the unparalleled quality of Medical Meditation. Quite simply, it succeeds where other forms of meditation fail. Because of this inherent success, there has recently been a grassroots, word-of-mouth movement among the public toward advanced meditation. This approach is much more popular than it was even ten years ago, as is evidenced by increasing enrollment in classes that involve kundalini yoga where Medical Meditation is taught. Also, more books and articles on the subject are in print than ever before, although almost all of them until now have been printed by small specialty publishing houses.

Medical Meditation surpasses the more mundane forms of meditation, I believe, because it more fully addresses every element of our physical and ethereal makeup. It is, to put it plainly, a more full-service approach. It nurtures every aspect of our being.

Medical Meditation

So what exactly is Medical Meditation? It is one of the newest and most cutting-edge advances in the field of integrative medicine. Medical Meditation is the use of advanced meditative techniques in a modern clinical setting. During approximately twenty-five years of medical practice—in which I have specialized in the areas of anesthesiology, pain management, brain regeneration, and integrative medicine—I have adapted and refined the use of kundalini yoga, combined with meditation, as a modality that I refer to as Medical Meditation.

Medical Meditation is not the simple, word-based meditation used to elicit the relaxation response. That type of therapy can be very helpful, and is widely practiced. But it is, in effect, the kindergarten version of Medical Meditation.

Medical Meditation uses advanced meditations, which consist of these unique attributes:

1. specific breathing patterns;
2. special postures and movements, including exact positioning of the hands and fingers;
3. particular mantras, consisting of distinct, vibratory sounds; and
4. a unique mental focus.

These various attributes fully involve the mind, body, and spirit of the meditator. The combination of all of the attributes exerts a synergistic effect, and endows Medical Meditation with far more power than standard meditation, which often involves simply relaxing.

Because there are so many variables in each Medical Meditation, there are dozens of different Medical Meditations, for a wide variety of medical conditions and illnesses. I have adapted each of these Medical Meditations from ancient advanced meditations that were employed for healing long before the advent of modern medicine. I combine Medical Meditation with the best modern medical techniques.

Each Medical Meditation has a specific physiological effect. There are specific Medical Meditations for arthritis, for heart disease, for AIDS, for cancer, for migraines, for asthma—and for nervous system regeneration. All of these I will share with you.

The clinical precision of Medical Meditation is extraordinary, and is simply not present in standard meditation. Make no mistake: standard meditation is extremely valuable in medical treatment. It has helped effect many recoveries from serious illnesses, when used as an adjunctive therapy, and sometimes even as a stand-alone therapy. Furthermore, standard meditation has a long history of clinical research, and has been studied by modern clinicians far more than Medical Meditation. Nonetheless, in my clinical practice, I have employed both standard meditation and Medical Meditation, and have found Medical Meditation to be considerably more powerful, and more predictable.

The greatest advantage of Medical Meditation is its specificity. Because Medical Meditation channels healing energy so precisely, each meditation has a sharp focus. Each is a veritable knifepoint of healing power. Each Medical Meditation solves a distinct, specific problem by bringing energy to targeted organs, glands, and systems, and also to the specific areas of the ethereal body, known as the chakras.

Some researchers believe that the ethereal body can bring healing power to the physical body, and that the physical body can bring healing power to the ethereal body. But even this view, I feel, imposes an artificial distinction. I see no barriers, nor any contradictions, between the physical and ethereal. We are all one, in body, mind, and spirit. We are all physical beings, and we are all ethereal beings. Medical Meditation treats us as such.

CHAPTER TWO

Healing the Physical
and Ethereal Bodies

How Medical Meditation Works

The Physical Milieu of the Body

As mankind emerged from the superstition of the Dark Ages into the rational world of the Renaissance, a hero of the intellect emerged whose indelible stamp still remains. It was René Descartes, who as a young man might have felt quite at home with the rebels of today, and who was one of the original bad boys of modern science. In his book *Discourse on Method,* his quintessential "portrait of the artist as a young punk," he lashes out at blind faith in all authorities, theological as well as intellectual. Every bit as radical as Galileo, who was arrested for his heresy, Descartes in his skepticism swept aside every assumption of the day, until he finally was left with the one fact he thought was provable: that he existed. As he put it, "I think, therefore I am." The beautiful simplicity of this statement has captivated modern thought ever since.

To arrive at this hard kernel of wisdom, Descartes used the method of reasoning known as deductivism: reasoning from a general set of facts to one specific, irrefutable fact. In so doing, Descartes elevated deductivism to a veritable religion of the intellect. Ever since, science has been based on deducing truth by breaking it down, reducing and separating each element until only certainty remains. In fact, Descartes even had his name attached to the principle: reductionist Cartesian thought.

Among the separate, unconnected entities that fascinated Descartes were: mind and spirit; mind and body; and body and spirit. They're separate, he insisted, and to lump them together is a travesty of old-fashioned, idol-worshiping superstition.

Descartes, a brilliant mathematician who brought algebra and geometry together as analytical geometry, claimed to be an expert only in the physical realm, not the spiritual. However, he intimated that only the physical world really mattered when he proclaimed that if he, like God, had been endowed with mastery over matter and space, he could have constructed the universe himself.

Modern medicine has been, until quite recently, absolutely dominated by reductionist Cartesian thought. Western doctors generally try to reduce a patient's pathology to a single, isolated cause. They then usually try to treat this pathology with a single, isolated modality. Furthermore, they tend to see problems as existing only in a single, separate organ or system at any one time.

Because of this reductivist approach, doctors are now for the most part classified in terms of their specialties. Even doctors who practice general medicine are now often classified as family practitioner specialists.

On one level, this appears to be reasonable.

There's only one problem with it. It doesn't work.

Virtually all of the latest scientific research indicates that each of the body's organs and systems is inextricably linked, often through connections so elegant and esoteric that they escaped scientific notice until just the past few years. For example, progress in advanced imaging techniques, as well as new biochemical research, has revealed connections between the hormonal, immunological, and gastrointestinal systems that were considered nonexistent ten years ago.

If Descartes were alive today, he might be a Young Turk professor somewhere, screaming, "Wake up and smell the holism! When evidence changes, change with it! And for God's sake, don't trust anybody over 300!"

Some of the most compelling research on the body's physical interrelationships, and also on the mind-body-spirit link, has come from the erudite Candace Pert, Ph.D., who was one of the discoverers of the endorphin system.

Dr. Pert has recently published fascinating research on the biochemical connections that knit the human being together. She has conclusively proved that the body contains an extraordinary system of receptors, tiny sensing devices that receive messages from specific chemicals, such as hormones and neurotransmitters. Until just the last few years, the allegory used to express the linkage between receptors and their specific chemicals was that of a biochemical lock and key. But Dr. Pert and others have shown that this mechanical concept is just not how it really works. Instead, receptors attach to their intended chemicals by sharing the same, distinct molecular vibration. This lends credence, I think, to the assumption of the ancient yoga masters—and modern quantum physicists—that vibration is integral to biological function.

The chemicals that attach to receptors are called ligands, from the Latin word *ligandus*, "that which bonds." The three types of ligands are: hormones, neurotransmitters, and peptides (or combinations of amino acids).

For many years, scientists thought that the ligand-receptor system was confined primarily to the nervous system, including the brain. Neurotransmitters, for example, were considered to be the chemicals of thought, and little else. But this isn't true. The exciting new evidence is that ligands and receptors are distributed throughout the body—and this changes the whole perception of the human mind, as we once knew it. It means, quite simply, that your mind is not just in your brain.

It means that throughout your body, there are chemicals of thought and emotion—what Dr. Pert calls information molecules. These molecules affect the way you feel, and how you think. In fact, Dr. Pert calls this ubiquitous system of molecules the second nervous system. She has shown that the body-mind connection is not, as previously believed, an exclusively electrical communication system, governed by the firings of nerve cells. It's also chemical: tangible, constant, and open to manipulation.

The brain is the focal point for thought and feeling, but amazingly, it's not the single site of the psyche. There are so-called hot spots or nodal points, saturated with receptors, throughout the body, where huge amounts of information come together and are processed. These nodal points in effect decide what messages to send to the brain for further processing, and what to ignore. The nodal points even have their own type of memory. In effect, each of them has a mind of its own. Many researchers think that these dispersed nodal-point mini-minds, so to speak, may be part of what we have long called the subconscious.

The discovery of this ligand-receptor system, with its powerful nodal points, proves that the mind-body connection isn't the one-way street, traveling from brain to body, long assumed. It's bidirectional. Chemically encoded information, or thought, travels from body to brain just as certainly as it travels from brain to body. As Dr. Pert writes in the eloquent *Molecules of Emotion,* "Mind doesn't dominate body, it becomes body—body and mind are one."

Since thought can exist as a physical entity—a molecule of information—memory too must partly exist as a solid, physical entity rather than just as a pattern of electrical firing of neurons, as long presumed. This may explain the existence of what we call instinct: the ability of a newborn creature to know things about its environment without having learned them. The newborn creature must, in a physical way, be hard-wired with the memory. This may also account for the phenomenon that some researchers have called cellular memory—the inborn fear of things like snakes and rats that so many people have.

The physical existence of memory may, in addition, explain the outcome of one of the most interesting experiments I've ever heard about. This experiment involved one of the most primitive forms of life, a type of worm called planaria. Scientists kept a group of planaria in a dark box, flashed a light at them, then shocked them with electricity. Over time the worms learned to coil into balls when they saw the light, in anticipation of the electric shock. Then the scientists ground up this group of worms and fed them to a new group of worms. They then flashed a light at the new group. The worms coiled into balls! They apparently had learned by eating a memory.

The implication of the physical existence of thought and memory, throughout the body, is profound. It means, for one thing, that the physical elements of Medical Meditation can alter thought and emotion. And it means that the mental elements can alter the body.

On a very practical level, it means that the immune system may be able to actually learn. This learning now appears not to occur in a mechanical way, the way a computer learns; instead this learning may well occur in much the same way that the psyche learns, through textures and variations of experience.

Furthermore, it may be that the brain can actually speak to the nodal points of the immune system, in a "language" that both understand. If this is true, and I suspect it is, it means that the body is so utterly competent and sophisticated that it is practically magical. In future years scientists may be better able to decode the language of the body and excise some of the mystery from this magic—just as Renaissance scientists like Galileo explained why the sun rose each day, thus draining the mystery from that previously magical occurrence.

My colleague Deepak Chopra, M.D., wrote eloquently of the language of the body in *Quantum Healing:* "Outfitted with a vocabulary to mirror the nervous system in its complexity, the immune system apparently sends and receives messages that are just as diverse. In fact, if being happy, sad, thoughtful, excited, and so on all require the production of neuropeptides and neurotransmitters in our brain cells, then the immune cells must also be happy, sad, thoughtful, excited—indeed, they must be able to express the full range of 'words' that neurons do."

The language of the body, of course, could not literally be verbal, but would be a much more fundamental form of communication. For example, in one experiment, researchers gave dogs an immune-suppressant drug, sweetened with saccharin. The drug, of course, lowered the dogs' immune function. Then the researchers gave the dogs just saccharin, and this too lowered their immunity. Thus, without having any conscious knowledge of what was happening, the dogs regulated their own immunity, using their own nonverbal, subconscious mind-body powers. They didn't talk themselves into lowered immunity. Nonetheless, an undeniable form of communication occurred between their brains and their bodies.

The amazing ability of the body to communicate gives new, rich meaning to the phrase "the wisdom of the body," which stress research pioneer Walter Cannon coined a century ago. Because actual thought appears to occur in the body, it also means that strictly physical activities can profoundly alter our thought patterns. For example, very recent research has shown that the simple act of breathing can change the type and quantity of peptides produced by the brain stem. All of the peptides in existence are now known to be present in the respiratory system, and this is probably the biological explanation for why something as simple as deep breathing can so effectively and predictably calm the mind, or in some people help release grief, fear, or anger.

We now know that molecules of emotion can literally be stored away in the body, just as surely as you store soup in your cupboard. When these molecules are released, and finally begin to circulate, they can allow people to feel emotions that had long been stored away. This commonly occurs when patients do breath work. They frequently feel an onrush of emotion—for no logical reason—and then often associate these emotions with long-buried memories.

Unfortunately, though, there is also a dark side to the physical existence of thought and emotion. When you subject your body to negative physical forces, they can cause you to feel negative emotions. Many people, in trying to understand why they feel bad, look for something or someone to blame. Frequently, though, this is just fruitless scapegoat thinking. It's quite possible that no one and no thing is to blame—except for negative physical forces that may be too subtle to notice. For example, because the upper intestine is so dense with receptors, I believe that negative forces that affect the gut can harm emotional homeostasis. Consider the word *dyspeptic*. It has two primary meanings. The first, according to the *New World Dictionary,* is "gloomy, or grouchy." The second is "the condition of impaired digestion." This indirectly infers, I believe, the connection that exists between impaired digestion and mood. Of course, it can be uncomfortable to have a digestive problem, and this could affect one's mood. But I don't believe the situation is always quite that simple. Patients with chronic heartburn, for example, have mentioned that heartburn really bothers their mood, far out of proportion to the actual discomfort it causes. This anecdotal evidence is by no means conclusive, of course, but I do think it's indicative of one of the many mind-body connections that we're finally beginning to understand.

Here's another interesting example of the interplay between the body and the emotions. The same receptor that attaches to the happiness neurotransmitter norepinephrine also attaches to viruses. Therefore, if a virus gets attached first, there may be no more room on the receptor for norepinephrine. But if norepinephrine gets there first, there may be no way for a virus to become attached to the receptor. Perhaps this explains why people suffering from a viral illness often complain of emotional malaise, above and beyond that caused by the discomfort of the illness. Some patients colloquially refer to this as their blah feeling, and say that it's a distinct, discrete emotional feeling, separate from the natural annoyance they feel from being sick. In fact, some patients who suffer from recurring, systemic viral involvement can accurately predict the onset of viral symptoms by noting a sudden decline in their moods. First they become anxious and depressed, for no apparent reason, and then they soon develop physical symptoms.

This same phenomenon may also explain why happiness and excitement so often seem to confer a degree of immunity from illness. As Candace Pert notes, "I never get sick when I'm about to go skiing!"

Similarly, one patient with chronic fatigue syndrome has frequently recovered from episodes of the illness by going skiing. The first several times that this occurred, the patient credited his recovery to the clean, fresh mountain air. This never made much sense to me, though. While it's true that fresh air is good for you, I've never heard of it curing an illness so quickly. Besides, it is clinically paradoxical for someone to recover from chronic fatigue symptoms through exercise, which generally exacerbates chronic fatigue syndrome. However, the patient then noticed that the same thing often occurred in the summer, when he went water-skiing in his boat. This led him to believe that the essential healing element was simply engaging in a joyful, exciting experience.

Many conventional doctors would dismiss this patient's frequent recoveries as meaningless, despite their regularity and predictability, two of the hallmarks of scientific investigation. These skeptical physicians would doubtless say that these recoveries represented only the placebo effect.

I see it quite differently. I refer to the mental power that can heal as the mind-power effect. The mind-power effect is one of the greatest forces in medicine. The mind-power effect cannot only heal by itself, but also makes effective physical therapies and medications more effective. For example, you would be more likely to recover from an illness if you knew you were receiving an effective drug than you would be if you received the same effective drug, but didn't know it.

The mind-power effect is most effective in patients who have positive outlooks, and who are responsive to the power of suggestion. Generally, patients who respond well to sham drugs also respond well to effective drugs. For example, in one study, a group of patients who had responded well to a sham drug responded with a 95 percent relief rate to an effective drug. However, another group of patients, who had not responded well to the sham drug, experienced only a 50 percent relief rate from the effective drug.

In the same way, drugs and surgeries that are later proven to be relatively ineffective tend to work well in the early stages of their use, before patients and doctors lose faith in them. In one study, surgeries that were later proven ineffective enjoyed an early success rate of 70 percent. There's an adage in medicine that says, "You should use drugs when they first come out, while they still work."

On the other hand, it's also quite possible to talk yourself into being sick with the nocebo effect, which is the opposite of the positive, mind-power effect. *Nocebo* is Latin for "I will cause pain." A study published in the *Journal of the American Medical Association* showed how strong the nocebo effect can be. A group of chronic pain patients were given a harmless sham drug and were told that it would help. Many of the patients were helped. However, 19 percent of the patients, apparently tired of false hope and failed therapies, refused to believe that anything could stop their pain, and reported that the harmless medication had made their pain worse. Some of them said it had made their pain permanently worse, even after they'd been told it had been a harmless substance.

Not just people with existing problems suffer from the nocebo effect. In one study, a group of students was told that a mild electric current would be sent through their brains, and that it might cause a headache in some of them. They were fitted with electrodes, but no electricity was applied. Even so, 70 percent of them suffered headaches.

It's well accepted among doctors that approximately 30 percent of patients experience the mind-power effect. But even that's not true. The 30 percent figure was derived from just one study, done in 1955. Researchers surveying much more recent studies on the mind-power effect have found that it's vastly more powerful than previously believed. The most commonly cited figure among the newer studies was an effectiveness rate of 70 percent, and in one study it reached 90 percent.

This is incredibly encouraging. It indicates that the mind-power effect is approximately as efficacious as some of the best medications and procedures in modern medicine. Truly, your mind—including your many nodal-point mini-minds—has the power to heal.

Some of the more progressive doctors, particularly those who practice integrative medicine, strive actively to exert the mind-power effect. Virtually all of them, though, enlist only the power of their patients' thoughts in their clinical efforts. With the advent of Medical Meditation, though, I believe that I have brought mind-power medicine to the next logical level.

With Medical Meditation, which precisely creates the mix of molecules of information for healing, the mind heals the body, and the body heals the mind. At the same time, the physical body heals the ethereal body, and the ethereal body heals the physical body. And the spirit—the divine spirit as well as the human spirit—pervades this entire healing milieu, adding a depth and a power that infuse the body and the mind with a healing force that no illness can withstand.

This healing force simply cannot be explained in dross physical terms—

in terms of matter and molecules. To have any true or workable knowledge of this healing force, we must go beyond the physical, into the ethereal.

The Realm of the Spirit

Long before modern science described our bodies in strictly physical terms, ancient healers described the body with an allegorical language that parallels the language of modern anatomical science. This ancient description of the body was based on our physical structure, but was phrased in ethereal terms. Among the key concepts of this perception of reality were the eight chakras, the nadis, and the five tattwas. These descriptions of the body may sound arcane, but as you'll soon note, they reflect our own modern physical descriptions.

THE EIGHT CHAKRAS

The *chakras* are our ethereal centers of consciousness and communication. Because *chakra* means "wheel," the energy in the chakras is often perceived as a swirling vortex, which is the most powerful physical force in nature, existing in events such as tornadoes and hurricanes. The chakras are swirled by polarized, opposing forces, just as tornadoes are formed by the clash of warm and cold air.

The chakras emanate from the center of the spinal cord and are the ethereal components of our physical nerve plexuses, organs, and glands. The chakras are considered to be centers of transformation. They interact with our thoughts, emotions, health, and physical functions. They exchange energy bidirectionally, from physical to ethereal, and ethereal to physical. They are believed to be the doorways of consciousness.

All eight chakras, or energy centers, are sacred and vital. This includes the lower chakras. However, to achieve the fullest experience of being, and to maintain full contact with the energy that surrounds us, it is important for energies to rise from the lower chakras, near the base of the spine, to the highest chakras, in and above the head. This allows our energies to meet and mingle with the energies of the cosmos, and it allows cosmic energy to return to our bodies.

- **The first chakra** (the *muladhara*) is located near the rectum and governs survival and self-destruction. It deals with our sense of tribalism, or family. It is powered by the polarity of bad and good.
- **The second chakra** (the *svadhistana*) is located in the pelvic area, and includes the sex organs. It reflects creativity and rejuvenation. The polarity from which it derives energy is the tension between projection and withdrawal. This chakra is the site of emotions about money, sex, and power.
- **The third chakra** (the *manipura*) is located at the navel, and focuses on personal identity, power, and judgment. The polarity expressed here is between fear and being. The chakra's physical connection is to the stomach, intestines, adrenals, kidneys, and pancreas.
- **The fourth chakra** (the *anahata*) is near the heart, and is the center of compassion and forgiveness. Here, the polarity that swirls the vortex is between giving and receiving. An imbalance here can cause cardiovascular and lung problems. It can also cause immune dysfunction, because the thymus is located in the fourth chakra.
- **The fifth chakra** (the *visuddha*) is near the throat, and is the arena of knowledge, truth, and willpower. It is appropriate, I believe, that the seat of the will should lie between the heart and the head. Problems here can be manifested physically as thyroid dysfunction, or as throat problems.
- **The sixth chakra** (the *ajna*) is located between the eyebrows, and is sometimes called the third eye. This is the center of discovery. This chakra sees what the other two eyes cannot see. Disturbances of this chakra, and also of the seventh chakra, can produce mental illness and cognitive disorders, as well as problems with the eyes, pituitary, pineal, and ears.
- **The seventh chakra** (the *sahashara*) is located at the top of the head, and connects the human being to the infinite. It is the entry point of the energy of the highest self. It is the exit point of personal energy.
- **The eighth chakra** (the *aura*) is located in the magnetic field generated by human life. The quality of the aura reflects the relative well-being of the person projecting it. The eighth chakra is

surrounded by the arc line, the body's first line of defense against illness. In much of the existing spiritual literature of healing, the eighth chakra is never mentioned. This, in my opinion, is a glaring error, which not only reduces understanding of the human condition but can also subvert a medical outcome when spiritual healing is applied.

Medical Meditations focus upon the specific chakras that are connected to the areas of distress. For example, the Medical Meditation for a heart condition would likely focus on the heart center, or fourth chakra. It would deliver healing energy, and resolve dysfunction that may have begun there as imbalanced polarity.

At other times, Medical Meditations transfer energy from one chakra to a higher one, if there is evidence that energy has become "stuck" at a given chakra. For example, one female patient had a severe energy blockage in her lower chakras, and this had apparently contributed to her devastating case of chronic fatigue syndrome. She'd had flu-like symptoms for two years, with muscle pain, fatigue, anxiety, blurred vision, and short duration of energy. The most common spiritual component of chronic fatigue syndrome is the perception of the patients that they are not living their own lives, but are trapped by the demands of others. In this case, the patient wanted to be an artist but was instead a lawyer, largely because of family expectations. As a result, her creative energy was not flowing out of the top of her head, but was stuck in her first chakra—her family chakra. When she began a program of Medical Meditation, this blocked energy began to flow much more freely, and she staged a dramatic recovery. This healing action did not solve the real-life conflict she faced, but it did halt the manifestation of this conflict in her physical body, as would any proper medical therapy. After she became free of illness, she finally became strong enough to resolve her career ambivalence.

Of course, her treatment included an obviously esoteric medical approach, which many physicians might have disdained. Many doctors would have simply prescribed counseling. By comparison, however, when the field of psychology was first explored in the nineteenth century, most of the doctors of that day considered it arcane, esoteric, and of no consequence to the health of the physical body. With hindsight, we can see that perspective was far too narrow.

THE NADIS

The *nadis* are a series of nonphysical energy conduits that connect the chakras, and reach out to the entire body, bringing energy and communication to the whole system. The nadis are somewhat like the nonphysical acupuncture meridians, which also carry energy and communication to the body. However, there are only 12 acupuncture meridians, while there are approximately 72,000 nadis. The nadis are sometimes considered to be the ethereal counterpart of the body's vast network of peripheral nerves, and appear to function in concert with them. They may also be associated with the nodal-point hot spots of receptors and ligands, the so-called second nervous system.

For centuries healers used the nadis to influence health, without any solid evidence that the nadis actually existed. Very recently, however, researchers verified the existence of these fluidlike energy channels, with the use of sophisticated radioactive scanning methods.

The nadis appear to physically affect the nature and quality of nerve transmission from the brain and spinal cord to the outlying peripheral nerves. Therefore, energy blockage among the nadis seems to be associated with pathological changes in the nervous system, and with the closely associated endocrine and immune systems. For example, a decreased flow of energy through the nadis to the throat chakra might result in decreased energy to the thyroid. The physical manifestation of this might be hypothyroidism.

Three nadis are of particular importance, because they are connected to the brain's limbic system, which controls memory and emotion. It also coordinates the functions of the hypothalamus, and helps control the endocrine system's master gland, the pituitary. These three nadis, the *ida*, *pingala*, and *shushmana*, have a tremendously important effect on the body's biochemistry.

THE FIVE TATTWAS

The five tattwas are the full, complete relationship that exists between personality, emotions, and illness. In essence, they are the big picture of a person's chakras and nadis.

The five tattwas are based upon five of the most primal desires: greed, lust, anger, pride, and attachment. Each tattwa endows the body with a vital energy that the body cannot live without. Without these energies, a person would, quite simply, be less than human.

If the energy inspired by the five tattwas is allowed to be unexamined and uncontrolled, a person will wallow in the most base condition of the tattwas, feeling lustful, greedy, and vain. But if the five tattwas are examined and cultured through the fine lens of meditation, these five human qualities can be experienced in their richest form, as love, ambition, and devotion. It is said that if the tattwas are "drunk from the cup of consciousness," a person can become one with God. As my own teacher, Yogi Bhajan, has written:

> Be greedy, that the end may be noble.
> Be lustful to live like God.
> Be angry at your own weakness.
> Be attached to the Divine Path.
> Be proud of God's grace.

The five tattwas can become imbalanced. If this becomes pronounced, it can markedly deter natural healing. I observed this once in a patient with severe liver disease. The patient was absolutely obsessed with her attachments, and couldn't bear the thought of letting go of anything, including her maturing children, her diminishing funds, her job, and certainly not her life. Her prognosis was dim, and a liver transplant was deemed unavoidable.

However, she was given a Medical Meditation that helped to balance her desperate need for attachment, and to better understand it. It worked wonders. Using just this Medical Meditation—along with a diet of rice, mung beans, daikon radishes, and beets—she experienced a complete recovery in three months, and did not require a transplant.

When this happened, she was radiantly happy and extremely relieved. She remarked, "I can hardly believe this happened. And I have no idea how it happened."

Truth be told, I'm not absolutely certain myself how it happened. Miraculous healing is always mysterious; otherwise, it wouldn't be a miracle. But I certainly have theories on how it happened.

Here's what I think.

How Medical Meditation Works

Medical Meditation works by directly impacting both the body's physical and ethereal milieus. It brings adaptability and regeneration to both of these aspects of our being. Furthermore, it helps the ethereal milieu to reinforce physical health, and it helps the physical milieu to reinforce ethereal health.

It achieves this, as I mentioned earlier, through the powerful effects of: (1) breath; (2) posture and movement, including finger positions; (3) mantras; and (4) mental focus.

BREATH

Breath creates movement, pulsation, vibration, and life. With breath, we bring some of the outer world into us, and we release some of ourselves into the world. The word *spirit* comes from the Latin *spiritus,* "breath."

Almost everyone knows that breathing slowly and deeply can help the mind relax. This is the most obvious effect of therapeutic breathing, but there are a great many more subtle effects. For example, breathing in quick abdominal breaths—the Breath of Fire—stimulates the splanchnic nerves in the abdominal cavity, and potentiates release of stimulating epinephrine and norepinephrine. It also produces an alpha and beta wave condition in the brain. Therefore, breathing in this manner can simultaneously create increased calmness and heightened alertness.

Other breathing techniques create a wide variety of physical effects. Breathing through the left nostril, for example, subtly stimulates activity in the right hemisphere of the brain's cortex, and can improve the functions of the brain that are most associated with that hemisphere, such as spatial reasoning. Breathing through the left nostril also produces a profound state of relaxation.

The breathing component of Medical Meditation can also help to focus energy upon particular chakras, and improve the quality of the five tattwas. One of my patients whose recovery was most notably tied to breath control was, as you might imagine, a person with a breathing disorder, asthma. This patient often had asthma attacks in response to stress, and I felt that she harbored a deep-seated sense of fear. I taught her the

Breath Meditation to Release Fear, and it had a remarkable effect. It decreased her underlying sense of fear, and halted chronic secretion of the chemicals that cause basal bronchial constriction. She gradually stopped using all of her medications. That was six years ago. Her asthma has never returned, and she still practices Medical Meditation.

POSTURE AND MOVEMENT

Posture and movement are the most outwardly visible aspects of Medical Meditation, and are vitally important. The postures and movements of Medical Meditation are primarily derived from kundalini yoga. Yoga is the ancient physical practice that joins the mind, body, and spirit. In fact, *yoga* means "to yoke, or join." Kundalini yoga unites one's essential being with the divine spirit, and also increases, channels, and balances the healing kundalini energy.

The primary effect of posture and movement is to enhance the flow of kundalini energy. The secondary effect is to increase and channel blood circulation. As a rule, kundalini energy and blood are both sent to the same distressed area. For example, when kundalini energy is channeled to the topmost crown chakra, blood is channeled to the brain. In this manner, the ethereal body and the physical body are both nurtured.

Very often, the goal of posture and movement is to send physical and nonphysical energy to a particular gland of the endocrine system, or a particular organ. For example, Medical Meditations use postures and movements that channel energy to the brain, the pituitary, the heart, the adrenals, and the lungs. Because energy can be directed with this degree of specificity, Medical Meditation can effectively focus primarily on the part of the body that most needs to be healed. Posture and movement, however, can also be used to exert generalized effects. For example, when your adrenals are stimulated, your entire body is energized, and your mood improves.

Posture and movement also help the body to remain supple and flexible. As you may remember, one of the primary goals of the Eastern approach is to help people adapt to the ever-present force of change, since change can be terribly destructive if a person doesn't adapt to it. The best way to adapt to change is to remain flexible. This is true figuratively, but also literally. In the Eastern philosophy, there isn't much difference between the figurative and the literal—both are considered equally real. Therefore, physical flexibility is highly prized in Oriental medicine. In some Asian cultures, a person's age is measured not only in years, but also in terms of physical flexibility.

One of my patients who benefited immensely from the postures and movements of his Medical Meditation was a young man who had suffered a crippling back injury, due to a fall from an oil rig. He was in constant pain, was on a smorgasbord of medications, and was unable to be physically active.

A few months of Medical Meditation changed his life. He first overcame his chronic pain, then began rebuilding the muscles, tendons, and ligaments that had been ripped apart by the fall. This man had unsuccessfully tried just about every other type of medical therapy, including a course of standard meditation. The meditation he tried, however, was ordinary sit-and-think meditation, and it had been a complete failure. This man was grossly impaired—biochemically, structurally, and emotionally—and he needed the "full-service" approach that only Medical Meditation offers.

HAND AND FINGER POSITIONS. Hand and finger positions are a vital element of the body's posture and movements. Their significance has not been isolated and studied nearly as much as the other aspects of Medical Meditation, but I am convinced by my own personal experience as a meditator and as a doctor that they are important.

From our study of anatomical science, we now know that the hands and fingers are highly represented in the brain; if you watched a PET scan of someone moving his or her fingers into different positions, you would see many areas of the brain light up. This indicates that various finger movements have a direct impact upon brain function.

We also know now that certain movements of the hands and fingers help the brain to pattern physical coordination. For example, it was recently shown in a study that children who took a few months of piano lessons improved significantly in their mathematical ability. A report published in March 1999 in the *Journal of Neurological Research* cited a study in which children scored 27 percent higher in math tests after taking piano lessons. This phenomenon, dubbed the Mozart effect, was believed to stem primarily from the power of music to teach spatial-temporal reasoning. I believe, however, that some of the benefit is also derived simply from the changing hand positions that occur while playing the piano. These positions, I believe, help to hard-wire the brain for optimal function.

From the perspective of the yoga masters, each area of the hand helps to control a specific area of the brain. Eastern healers think that various discrete neurological effects can be gained by, for example, touching the fingertips to the thumb, or crossing certain fingers.

This aspect of Medical Meditation remains mysterious, but we will probably understand it better as technological medicine progresses. Six years ago, no one was familiar with the Mozart effect, and now it is widely known. Perhaps someday soon we will catch up to the wisdom of the ancient healers.

MANTRAS

Mantras are a powerful healing force, because of the vibratory effects of their sounds. If a tree falls in the forest and no one is there to hear it, does it make a sound? Of course not. It only makes a vibration. Sound only occurs when vibrations strike the eardrum and are carried to the brain. This is just a way of pointing out the fact that every sound is also a vibration. Particular vibrations can strongly stimulate the glands of the endocrine system, especially those located in the head and neck. This includes the pituitary, the system's master gland, as well as the hypothalamus.

Different mantras have markedly different effects upon the function of the endocrine system. In one interesting experiment at the University of

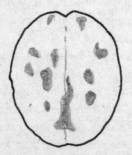
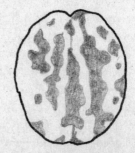

Before Medical Meditation   **After Medical Meditation**

The increased amount of dark areas in the second image indicates the improvement experienced by a meditator in oxygenation, blood flow, and glucose uptake in the brain.

Arizona, my colleague Gurucharan Singh Khalsa, Ph.D., observed brain function with a PET scan and noted that during the chanting of the mantra "Sa Ta Na Ma," there was a strong shift in brain activity to the right frontal and parietal regions. This shift indicated an improvement in mood and alertness.

It has also been shown that chanting certain yoga mantras stimulates the vagus nerve, the most important single nerve in the body. The vagus nerve, which travels through the neck near the jaw, services the heart, lungs, intestinal tract, and back muscles.

Sound currents also strongly influence the nadis and chakras by vibrating the upper palate of the mouth, which has eighty-four points connected to the body's ethereal energy system. Some of these points carry energy directly to the hypothalamus and to the pituitary. Striking these points on the palate with the tongue has been compared to striking the key of a computer with your finger—the act of striking is simple, but the effect can be profound.

One patient who seemed to benefit from the vibratory effects of sound currents was a young woman who had contracted HIV from her boyfriend. Her Medical Meditation was intended to increase immunity, in part by

Effects of Striking Meridian Points on Upper Palate

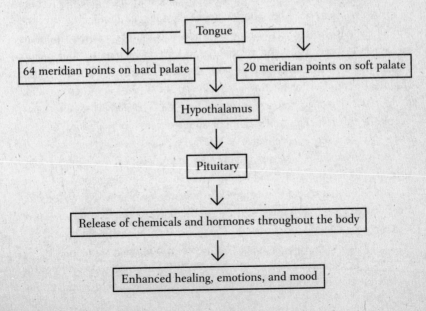

stimulating the immune system's thymus gland, via the pituitary, with sound vibrations. This naturalistic form of ultrasound seemed to have an almost immediate effect, judging from her white blood cell count. Using primarily Medical Meditation and nutritional therapy, the woman has remained virtually symptom-free for more than fifteen years. This result compares very favorably to even the best of the new pharmacological approaches.

MENTAL FOCUS

Mental focus is probably the most obvious of the five healing modalities that comprise Medical Meditation. It has long been recognized that a person's cognitive and emotional processes have a profound impact upon health. For the most part, this impact is mediated via the endocrine system.

When you meditate, your rational thought processes, housed in your cortex, begin a quiet dialogue with your brain's emotional centers, the hippocampus and amygdala, both of which are in your limbic system. When your cortex and limbic system agree that it is appropriate to relax, they relay the message to the hypothalamus, which connects the brain to the endocrine system. This releases a flood of calming neurotransmitters and hormones, which soothe the entire body. The immune system then secretes its own molecules of information, some of which return to the brain, helping to complete this circuitry of healing. You shift into a relaxed alpha brain wave pattern, and your nervous system is dominated by the inhibitory parasympathetic branch. When the parasympathetic nervous system is favored, you send relatively more nerve signals to your organs and glands of immunity, such as your thymus. As this occurs, you reach the ideal condition for healing—what mystics call the sacred space. One of my patients once remarked to me that the attitude of meditation—devoid of self-criticism and judgment about others—is really one of love. Thus, in a real sense, love heals.

As a physician, I have seen many amazing recoveries when people consistently reach this condition of elevated mental and emotional power. Often, the problems that respond most dramatically are slowly progressing degenerative diseases such as cancer and cardiovascular disease. The degenerative diseases are generally exacerbated by negative mental conditioning, and can be impacted successfully with positive mental conditioning.

One of my more recent experiences with positive mental conditioning involved a cancer patient. This person, a thirty-four-year-old woman, contracted breast cancer at the same time her public role model, Jacqueline Kennedy Onassis, contracted lymphoma. When she saw that Mrs. Onassis was dying, it shocked and disheartened her. The patient didn't see how she could survive if her hero couldn't, particularly since Mrs. Onassis had access to every possible medical resource. She was in despair, and sinking fast, according to her tests.

The patient was placed on a Medical Meditation program, along with medical therapy, that was designed to change her emotional outlook. The mantra devised for her was "Healthy am I, happy am I, holy am I." She was absolutely astounded to find that this simple meditation greatly improved her disposition. Having said the words, she began to believe them, and her belief was a powerful medicine. As she began to recover, her Medical Meditation was changed to one that released anger, and this further buoyed her spirits and resolve. This happened several years ago, and now the patient is cancer-free.

Obviously, I'm not claiming that this meditation cured the patient's cancer. But it did place her in the right frame of mind to fight her cancer effectively. I am convinced that her recovery could not have occurred without a change in her mental outlook.

Another important element of mental focus is simply focusing your attention on the particular area of your body that you wish to affect. For example, if you have a problem with your kidneys and are trying to send healing energy to them, you should focus on them during your meditation and visualize them becoming healthy. Or if you are trying to activate your sense of intuition during meditation, you should focus on your brow area, or third eye.

A simple exercise for using mental focus is to try to warm your cold hands or feet by focusing on them and imagining that they are becoming warmer. This simple action, which most people are able to achieve, warms the extremities by increasing blood flow to them.

SADHANA

When all of the elements of Medical Meditation are put together and practiced with regularity and enthusiasm, it constitutes a daily spiritual practice, or *sadhana*, pronounced "sod-na." Doing your daily sadhana is like putting money in your spiritual bank account. It not only helps relieve and reverse existing conditions but also prevents illness. Even more important, it is the key to spiritual realization and inner peace—which is the ultimate foundation of all health.

The best time to practice your sadhana is in the ambrosial hours of the early morning—the *amrit vela,* "time of nectar." This time, before the sun rises, is the stillest, sweetest time to be alive. This is also the time when the master hormones of the pituitary gland are secreted. Therefore, morning meditation can influence endocrinological secretions that will govern how you feel all day long. A recent study showed that when stress hormones are allowed to rise in the morning, it can increase susceptibility to stress-related illness, including cardiovascular disease and Alzheimer's disease. Sadhana also works so well because the exercises balance all the centers of ethereal energy, including the chakras.

Of course, it takes discipline to practice sadhana, but many people with serious problems are very well motivated. For example, one patient almost lost her leg in a riding accident, and was desperate to heal. Initially, her doctors had told her that her leg would have to be amputated, but she refused, so they reattached the leg, to the best of their capabilities. The reattachment worked, but her prognosis for walking again was extremely negative.

She began to practice the Medical Meditation to Heal Self and Others with great fervor, and almost never missed her morning sadhana. Incredibly, her leg regained its strength and physical integrity, and even her bones began to grow. She is now walking, and even rides horses again.

Once, when she was asked if she considered her morning sadhana to be an imposition, she just looked amused and incredulous. For the ill and injured, Medical Meditation is not a problem. It's a solution.

CHAPTER THREE

Scientific Research on Medical Meditation

Now let's analyze meditation as a healing modality, using just facts and figures, studies and experiments, charts and graphs. After all, Medical Meditation is based at least as much on rationalism as it is on spiritualism and intuition. It's important to remember that kundalini yoga, one of the foundations of Medical Meditation, is an ancient science, not a philosophy nor a religion. To be fully credible, Medical Meditation must withstand the scrutiny of the modern scientific method. Only by subjecting Medical Meditation to the rigors of science can we fully appreciate it.

Metaphorically, if Medical Meditation is a river of thought that has flowed from ancient days to ours, rationalism forms the banks of this river. Rationalism is the guiding, channeling force that gives this river of thought its power and shape. Without the strength and integrity of its banks, any river would become a formless stand of water, vulnerable to stagnation and evaporation. Earthen banks are the water's opposing force. Absent these seeming obstructions, there can be no river.

The Mind, the Brain, and the Body

To fully comprehend the power of Medical Meditation, we must have an understanding of its mechanism of action: how it works. In previous chapters, I've shown that Medical Meditation can help to open the channels of communication that exist between mind and body, in part by helping to link the brain with the body's nodal-point hot spots, which contain the neurotransmitters, hormones, and peptides that can speak the brain's own language. I've also shown that the psyche can directly influence the body, through the mind-power effect. Both of these powerful and fascinating actions involve a relatively new field of medicine called psychoneuroimmunology (PNI). Some doctors refer to this as psychoneuroendoimmunology, but most don't, simply because the word is too long. As the word itself indicates, this field of medicine links the psyche (psycho), the nervous system (neuro), the endocrine system (endocrinology), and the immune system (immunology). The basic theory of this medical approach is that the mind, brain, endocrine, and immune systems function in concert, to provide stable health in an ever-changing environment. The exciting premise of this field is that a person can intervene in any one of these four systems to improve the function of the other three, and restore health.

Intervention, unfortunately, seems to be quite necessary, because each of these three important elements of our being is under constant assault. Every single day, we must all endure a barrage of stress, toxic chemicals, viruses, bacteria, fatigue, and other insults. There is absolutely no way to escape biological assaults. Even the healthiest natural forces—sunshine and oxygen—cause damage. Sunshine subjects us to solar radiation, which damages the skin and lowers immunity, and oxygen produces cellular oxidation, which literally burns up cells from the inside out.

Perhaps the harshest of all physical assaults, though, comes simply from the passage of time. As time passes, minor damage mounts up, and cells, organs, and systems simply wear out.

One of the first systems that wears out is the endocrine system, the system of ductless glands that secretes hormones. Many researchers now believe, and I agree, that the primary reason we deteriorate as we age is due to the degeneration of the endocrine system. Furthermore, the function of the immune system generally follows the function of the endocrine system. This idea has been dubbed the neuroendocrine theory of aging by the esteemed Ward Dean, M.D., and others.

We usually think of old age as something that suddenly clamps down in our fifties, sixties, or seventies. But the newest research shows that this is not really how aging occurs. In fact, the primary characteristics of aging—organ decline, gland decline, and energy decline—begin at a much earlier age than previously believed. Most researchers now think that significant effects of aging begin as soon as a person's early twenties. At approximately this age, various glands of the endocrine system begin to decline, and to produce markedly fewer of the hormones that help keep us youthful and healthy. For example, the critically important hormone known as human growth hormone, or HGH, begins to drop off rapidly even before people reach age twenty. As early as age thirty, production of HGH has dropped to a fraction of what it was during its peak years, as the following chart indicates.

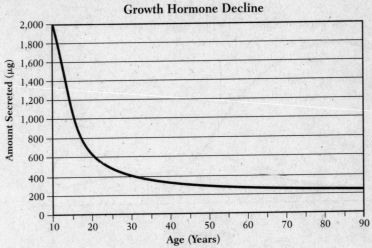

Growth Hormone Decline

Decline in secretion of growth hormone with age
Elderly levels are reached in most people by age 35-40 (Klatz, 1997)

The implications of this HGH decline are very disturbing; human growth hormone is vitally important in helping people to feel energetic, to repair their own muscles and other tissues, and to retain strong immunity.

Other endocrine glands are equally vulnerable. The pineal gland, which produces the sleep hormone melatonin, quickly declines with age, until it generally becomes calcified, and completely dysfunctional, in most elderly people. It's believed that this decline contributes significantly to the increase in sleep disorders that occurs with aging. Melatonin is also a powerful antioxidant and free-radical scavenger, so the decline of the pineal probably also contributes to an overall decrease in health.

Much of this endocrinological decline is cross-linked. For example, as melatonin declines, people get less deep, delta-wave sleep, and deep sleep is the time during which HGH is naturally released.

Another endocrine gland that declines precipitously with age is the thymus, the most important single gland of the immune system. The following chart clearly shows that as the aging thymus gland degenerates in size and function, illness increases.

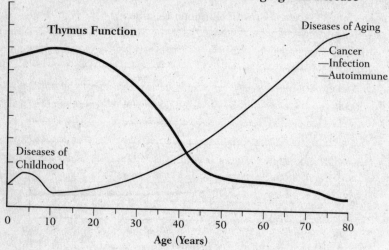

Relationship of Thymus Function to Aging and Disease

Similarly, the extremely important steroidal hormone DHEA (dehydroepiandrosterone) drops off considerably as we age, and this decline causes innumerable problems. DHEA helps protect the body from stress, and is vitally important for maintaining a good mood, a normal sex drive, a stable body-fat ratio, and a high level of energy. It also helps protect the brain from damage, since it is 6.5 times more concentrated in brain cells than in blood. In *Brain Longevity*, Cameron Stauth and I showed how low levels of DHEA can be one of the worst risk factors for Alzheimer's disease. One study we mentioned showed that Alzheimer's patients had only about half as much DHEA as healthy older people. In my own clinical practice, almost all of my Alzheimer's patients have low levels of DHEA.

Besides helping prevent Alzheimer's, proper DHEA levels dramatically improve general health. In one remarkable twelve-year study, men with the highest DHEA levels had the best health of any of the subjects being studied, even if they smoked and had high cholesterol. In this study, for every

20 percent increase in DHEA levels there was a 48 percent decrease in heart disease, and a 36 percent decrease in death from any cause.

One of the most important things DHEA does is to protect against the ravages of the stress hormone cortisol, which can be the single most damaging hormone in the body, if too much is secreted. High levels of cortisol drastically increase the incidence of Alzheimer's, cardiovascular disease, depression, chronic anxiety, and many other conditions and diseases.

The overall impact of endocrine decline is staggering. Dr. Ward Dean has shown that endocrine decline is implicated in the diseases that kill 85 percemt of all people. These include: (1) obesity, (2) atherosclerosis, (3) hypertension, (4) diabetes, (5) cancer, and (6) autoimmune disorders.

Dr. Dean and others believe that an essential reason that the endocrine system declines is because of the associated decline of the hypothalamus, the part of the brain that interfaces directly with the endocrine system. The hypothalamus receives its orders from the brain's amygdala—the emotional center of the brain, which is part of the limbic system. It then relays these orders to the pituitary gland, the master gland of the endocrine system.

The body depends on the hypothalamus to keep its systems in balance. It's up to the hypothalamus to order up more adrenaline, more thyroid hormones, more testosterone—whatever is needed to maintain proper balance in the body. This balance of the body's systems is often referred to as homeostasis. Helping the hypothalamus to maintain homeostasis is the pineal gland, the pea-shaped endocrine gland that is located near the forebrain. However, function of both the hypothalamus and the pineal decline with age. As you'll recall, the pineal may become totally nonfunctional in elderly people.

There are several reasons for this decline. One is simple wear and tear. The most exhausting aspect of this wear and tear is the stress response. The stress response, or fight-or-flight mechanism, occurs every time the brain perceives a threat. When that happens, the amygdala, in conjunction with the brain's cortex, demands that the hypothalamus take immediate action and order the secretion of extra stress hormones, including adrenaline and cortisol. When the secretions are sufficient, a feedback mechanism alerts the hypothalamus to shut off the supply. Over time, though, after considerable stress, this feedback mechanism deteriorates, and the hypothalamus simply becomes exhausted. In some people, this can be manifested as an inability to regain calmness after a threat has passed.

The stress response also hurts the hypothalamus by hurting the part of the brain that interfaces with the hypothalamus. This part of the brain, the limbic system, is harmed terribly by stress. The harm caused by stress to the limbic system (and especially the limbic system's hippocampus) is one of the leading causes of age-associated memory impairment and Alzheimer's. The hippocampus, in particular, is the most important single site in the brain for memory. When the stress hormone cortisol strikes the hippocampus, it destroys hippocampal cells. As I often say, repeatedly subjecting the hippocampus to high levels of cortisol is almost like bathing the brain in battery acid. Thus, we see another vicious spiral of decline: stress response/cortisol secretion/ hypothalamic decline/increased stress response.

Other factors that cause the hypothalamus to decline over time are: (1) reduced quantity of receptors for hypothalamic hormones, (2) fat accumulation on and around the hypothalamus, (3) cholesterol buildup in neurons, (4) a decline in the neurotransmitters the hypothalamus needs (such as serotonin), and (5) chronic insufficiency of glucose (for cognitive energy).

The end result is a degenerating body and brain that just don't adapt to change as well as they once did.

As the hypothalamus declines, it becomes far less adept at responding perfectly to minor imbalances. Sometimes it calls for the production of too few hormones, and sometimes too many. In effect, it loses its elasticity and flexibility.

As the hypothalamus and pituitary decline, they trigger declines in the rest of the endocrine system. Then, as the endocrine system declines, so do the body and the mind. Fat clings to the abdomen. Skin loses its suppleness. Memories fade. Viruses go unopposed. Eye muscles lose their ability to contract. Immunity wanes. Sex drive declines. Aging occurs.

Aging, though, is not the only problem caused by the decline of the endocrine system. The same factors that cause aging reduce quality of life, and health, in young people. You don't need to be old to have poor immunity, impaired eyesight, low energy, depression, insomnia, decreased sex drive, poor muscle tone, hypoglycemia, obesity, muscle pain, impaired cognitive function, or any other of the many problems associated with endocrine decline. These problems are more prevalent among the elderly, but are absolutely common among young people. Unfortunately, many of them appear to be increasingly common among young people. Two of the most obvious are depression and obesity, which are now at their highest rates in history among the young. Remember, old age doesn't suddenly swoop down at age sixty. Aging starts early, especially if you subject your body and brain to one physical and emotional assault after another.

Forever Young

By now, I imagine you're ready for some good news. I have some. There is a powerful mechanism that can ameliorate the ravages of aging and confer youthful vitality—at any age. That mechanism is Medical Meditation.

Medical Meditation, though, is not the only thing you can do to obviate endocrine decline. Several physical lifestyle elements are also quite important. The first is to eat a nutrient-dense diet, low in saturated fat. The second is to exercise, which helps restore hypothalamic sensitivity, increases production of growth hormone, and enhances hormonal balance. The third is to take specific nutrients that help your body to produce and regulate hormones, such as arginine (for human growth hormone), ginseng (which regulates stress hormones), and phosphatidyl serine (which increases hypothalamic health). Other nutrients that help the endocrine and nervous systems are ginkgo biloba; schizandra; acetyl L-carnitine; coenzyme Q-10; vitamins E and C; the minerals selenium, magnesium, and zinc; and omega-3 fatty acids, such as DHA and flaxseed oil. The fourth thing you can do is to engage in hormonal replacement therapy. This may include taking DHEA, melatonin, and other hormones. For women, it may also include taking estrogen. Recent research also indicates the value of hormone replacement therapy in men, with testosterone and growth hormone.

But engaging in these physical actions is less important than fighting the effects of endocrine decline at its very source, the glands themselves. Only one therapy can do this: Medical Meditation. Medical Meditation (and to a lesser degree, other forms of meditation) directly rejuvenates the hypothalamus, the pituitary, the pineal, and other endocrine glands. Think of it as endocrine exercise. In addition, Medical Meditation is also the single most effective countermeasure against the stress response. In fact, Dr. Herbert Benson named his meditative approach the relaxation response simply to indicate that it has the exact opposite biological effect as the stress response.

Every form of meditation helps control stress. However, medical studies indicate that some forms are more effective than others. Furthermore, it appears that some forms are significantly more powerful than others at directly rejuvenating the endocrine system. Medical Meditation seems to be notably more efficient than other forms of meditation at restoring endocrine health. The main reason for this is that Medical Meditation combines yoga and meditation. In fact, Medical Meditation employs a form of yoga that was specifically designed to improve endocrine function. The ancient yoga masters, of course, did not have modern anatomic knowledge of the endocrine system, but they did refer to it in their own ethereal language. For example, the third-eye chakra is located at exactly the same point as the pituitary gland. The throat chakra is located at the same point as the thyroid gland. As we delve deeper into the language of the ethereal, you will note that endless similarities exist between the physical body and the ethereal body.

Other forms of meditation do not address the endocrine system so directly, but still help stop stress. Among the many forms of meditation that do this are:

- Prayer
- Visualization
- Sufi meditation
- Guided imagery
- Mindfulness meditation
- The relaxation response
- Transcendental Meditation
- Zen Buddhist meditation
- Native American meditation
- Movement meditation, including t'ai chi and Qigong

The central, common element that all of these forms of meditation share is relaxation, with a suspension of thought, which causes the opposite physiological effect as the stress response. My favorite definition of this type of meditation is:

> *When thine eye is single, thy whole body also is full of light.*
>
> —Jesus of Nazareth

Similarly, there are also many forms of yoga, some of which can also be powerful forces for rejuvenating the endocrine system, and relieving stress. Among the most common types of yoga are:

- Karma yoga (serving others)
- Bhakti yoga (focusing on the love of God)
- Hatha yoga (achieving balance through physical postures)
- Raja yoga (which includes breathing, movement, and mental focus)
- Kundalini yoga (bringing energy and balance from the lower chakras to the higher, using breathing, movement, mental focus, hand positions, and mantras)

Of these forms of meditation and yoga, I believe that Medical Meditation, which combines meditation with all five of the elements of kundalini yoga, most effectively heals the body. As the most comprehensive, full-service form of meditation, it most effectively channels energy to specific glands and organs, and most effectively rejuvenates the endocrine system. It achieves this, in part, simply because of the long-standing, strong emphasis of kundalini yoga on endocrine function.

However, several forms of meditation other than Medical Meditation are quite popular in modern Western culture, and are of undeniable value. Let's now scientifically assess the most popular, common forms of meditation, and examine the medical studies that prove their effectiveness as viable medical modalities.

Studies on Meditation

Among the most objective and rigorous studies on meditation were those recently funded by the federal government's new Office of Alternative Medicine, or OAM. This agency, which is part of the National Institutes of Health, subjects alternative modalities to the same criteria used to analyze standard modalities. Much of the research cited in this section was produced under the auspices of the OAM.

According to the OAM's omnibus 1994 report on meditation, "over a period of 25 years, Benson and colleagues have developed a large body of research." Because of the research of Benson and others, says the report, "meditation in general and the relaxation response in specific have slowly moved from alternative to mainstream medicine, although they are still overlooked by many conventional doctors."

The research indicates that the relaxation response—in which meditators sit quietly, clear their minds, and focus on a calming phrase—achieves the following biological reactions: marked reduction in oxygen use; notably lower secretion of stress hormones; increase in immune factors, including blood leukocyte production; and calm brain-wave activity. These factors remain intact for several hours after this form of meditation ends.

As a result of the physical factors, meditators enjoyed improved health. Among the many improvements were the following:

- Premenstrual syndrome symptoms decreased by 57 percent.
- Migraine headaches decreased notably.
- Anxiety and depression were reduced significantly.
- Working people missed fewer work days due to illness.
- Patients with AIDS and cancer experienced decreased symptoms.
- Seventy-five percent of patients with insomnia were cured, and almost 25 percent improved.
- Patients with chronic pain required an average of 36 percent less treatment.
- Patients with high blood pressure recovered completely, or improved.

Guided Imagery, Autogenic Training, Biofeedback, and Progressive Relaxation

Besides the relaxation response, several other no-frills approaches to meditation have also gained scientific acceptance. They include guided imagery, autogenic training, biofeedback, and progressive relaxation. These approaches share the common goal of helping patients relax and consciously control their own autonomic functions, such as heartbeat and skin temperature.

Numerous well-conducted studies have shown that these approaches produce improvements in cardiovascular function, use of oxygen, blood glucose levels, reactivity to stressors, and immune function. For example, in one study of biofeedback, 25 percent of patients with high blood pressure were able to stop taking medication entirely, and even more patients were able to reduce use of medication.

I support the use of these modalities, and have often noted their clinical effectiveness. However, I believe they are essentially one-dimensional techniques that confer primarily just relaxation, rather than direct endocrine enhancement. Furthermore, they appear to have only a moderate ability to intervene in the flow of ethereal energy. Therefore, I do not rely upon these techniques, but have simply incorporated their best elements into Medical Meditation. For example, imagery can be a helpful aspect of Medical Meditation, because it helps the psyche to stop thinking in words. Furthermore, when your mind actively focuses on an image, it more fully involves the visualization-related temporal lobes, and reduces the degree of verbal static that is constantly bombarding the frontal lobe of the neural cortex.

MINDFULNESS MEDITATION

One of the most popular forms of meditation, mindfulness meditation, has also been validated by recent studies. In mindfulness meditation, the meditator does not concentrate on a specific mantra, image, or thought, but instead allows the mind to wander, while focusing upon the breath. As the mind wanders, though, the meditator strives for a heightened awareness of each passing thought and image. According to mindfulness expert Jon Kabat-Zinn, Ph.D., mindfulness means "learning how to stop all your doing and shift over to a 'being' mode."

Numerous experiments indicate that mindfulness meditation has profound physiological effects. For example, in one experiment, mindfulness meditation helped patients with moderate to severe psoriasis to clear their skin. When patients listened to a mindfulness meditation tape during treatment with ultraviolet light therapy, they recovered significantly faster and more completely than patients who received only treatment with ultraviolet light.

In another study, cancer patients were able to produce notably more melatonin than a control group of cancer patients when they engaged in mindfulness meditation. Melatonin production is an accurate marker of stress perception, so it is sensible to assume that the meditating patients experienced less stress than the nonmeditators. Because stress harms the immune response, it is reasonable to believe that stress mediators—such as mindfulness meditation, in this case—may prolong survival and heighten quality of life in some patients.

Mindfulness meditation has also been proven by studies to decrease panic attacks, decrease general anxiety, reduce levels of chronic pain, reduce incidence of headaches, improve response rates to drug and alcohol addiction treatment, and reduce obesity.

TRANSCENDENTAL MEDITATION

The Transcendental Meditation program is the most popular and most scientifically examined form of meditation in Western culture. As you may know, Transcendental Meditation is meditation in which a mantra is used.

The Transcendental Meditation program has been studied since the mid-1970s, and about 600 controlled studies have been published, many in peer-reviewed journals. According to the government's OAM report, the Transcendental Meditation program has been proven to achieve the following:

- Reduction of anxiety
- Reduction of chronic pain
- Lowered levels of cortisol
- Increase in cognitive function
- Reduction of substance abuse
- Lowered blood pressure
- Improvement in post-traumatic stress syndrome
- Reduction in use of medical care and hospitalization

Another fascinating study of the Transcendental Meditation program was one that measured biological age—how old a person is physiologically rather than chronologically. Determinants included blood pressure, vision, and hearing. As you can see, the long-term Transcendental Meditation program participants, who had been doing the Transcendental Meditation program for five or more years, were physiologically twelve years younger than their nonmeditating counterparts. Even the short-term participants were physiologically five years younger than the controls.

An even stronger study on aging and the Transcendental Meditation program, performed with greater methodological precision, was conducted by researchers at Harvard and published in the *Journal of Personality and Social Psychology* in 1989. This study analyzed elderly people who were introduced to the Transcendental Meditation program. In a short time they showed numerous beneficial changes, and ultimately lived longer, on average, than patients in a control group that did not practice the Transcendental Meditation program. The positive results were noted to endure when a follow-up study was conducted more than ten years later.

Another good study of general health, indicating overall health improvement in practitioners of the Transcendental Meditation program,

Reversal of the Aging Process
through the Transcendental Meditation Technique

Reversal of the Aging Process

The Transcendental Meditation technique is a major component of the Maharishi Vedic Approach to Health℠. This study examined the effect of the Transcendental Meditation Program on what researchers in the field of aging have called the "biological age" of a person—how old a person is physiologically in contrast to chronologically. As a group, long-term Transcendental Meditation Program participants, who had been practicing the Transcendental Meditation Program for more than five years, were physiologically 12 years younger than their chronological age, as measured by lower blood pressure, better near-point vision, and better auditory discrimination. Short-term Transcendental Meditation Program participants were physiologically 5 years younger than their chronological age. The study was statistically controlled for the effects of diet and exercise.

References: 1. International Journal of Neuroscience, 16 (1982); 53–58. 2. Journal of Personality and Social Psychology, 57 (1989); 950–964. 3. Journal of Behavioral Medicine (1986); 327–334. Reprinted with the permission of the Maharishi University of Management.

shows the decreased use of medical services. As this graph indicates, this health benefit was enjoyed by all ages, but was increasingly significant as aging occurred. It appears as if the antiaging effects of the Transcendental Meditation program result in notably less acute illness among older people on a day-to-day basis. This study tracked the health of 2,000 Transcendental Meditation practitioners over 5 years, and matched them against a similar, nonmeditating control group. The Transcendental Meditation group experienced a 56 percent lower rate of hospitalization for all causes, along with 87 percent less hospitalization for cardiovascular disease, 55 percent less hospitalization for cancer, and 87 percent less hospitalization for nervous system diseases.

The Transcendental Meditation program has long enjoyed a strong base of financial support, provided primarily by government and university research support. This revenue has been used, quite wisely, to build a body of research evidence on the Transcendental Meditation program. Other

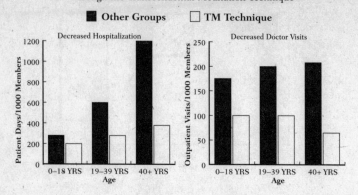

Decreased Hospitalization and Doctor Visits
Through the Transcendental Meditation Technique

■ Other Groups   □ TM Technique

A 5-year study of medical care utilization statistics on 2,000 people throughout the U.S. who regularly practiced the Transcendental Meditation Program found that their overall rate of hospitalization was 56% lower than the norm. The group practicing the Transcendental Meditation technique had fewer hospital admissions in all disease categories compared to the norm—including 87% less hospitalization for cardiovascular disease, 55% less for cancer, 87% less for diseases of the nervous system, and 73% less for nose, throat, and lung problems.

References: 1. Psychosomatic Medicine, 49 (1987); 493–507. 2. American Journal of Health Promotion, 19 (1996); 208–216. Reprinted with the permission of the Maharishi University of Management.

forms of meditation are not sold as a commercial product, however, and this has limited the funds that are available for their research. Partly because of this, other forms of meditation have been subjected to far fewer controlled studies than the Transcendental Meditation program.

Some studies and reports do exist, though, and more are under way. A recent fascinating article in the *New York Times* described a program in which patients at the influential Memorial Sloan-Kettering Cancer Center were taught a form of concentrative meditation. This report indicated clearly that patients experienced relief of pain, lowered blood pressure, decreased heart rate, improved mood, reduced anxiety, and increased cognitive function. The program prompted one observer, Dr. Woodson Merrell, of the Beth Israel Medical Center, to remark that meditation "is perhaps the most powerful tool for health."

MEDICAL MEDITATION

Several studies have compared the effectiveness of various forms of meditation. From this collection of studies, it appears as if the relaxation response is more effective than the least-involving forms of meditation, such as guided imagery or biofeedback. It also seems, however, that the relaxation response is rather less effective than nonconcentrative meditation, such as mindfulness meditation. The two forms of meditation that appear to be the most effective are the Transcendental Meditation program and Medical Meditation.

Using common sense as guide, Medical Meditation would prevail in most comparisons with Transcendental Meditation, simply because it combines two powerful approaches: meditation and yoga. As many studies support meditation as a healing modality, yoga is also well documented as biologically therapeutic. It has been successfully applied in a wide variety of conditions, including chronic pain, depression, cardiovascular disease, memory loss, lung disorders, cancer, gastrointestinal problems, arthritis, fibromyalgia, multiple sclerosis, and chronic fatigue syndrome.

One of the most fundamental tenets of integrative medicine is that a comprehensive approach, consisting of two or more synergistic modalities, is almost always more effective than a single, isolated approach. For example, in a recent study at Brigham and Women's Hospital, Medical Meditation was compared to basic meditation in regard to its effect upon the brain. This study was designed by my friend and colleague Gurucharan Singh Khalsa, Ph.D., one of the world's leading academic researchers on Medical Meditation, and conducted by Sara Lazar, Ph.D., of the Mind/Body Medical Institute through the Beth Israel Deaconess Hospital. This study disclosed that in basic meditation, only a small area of the brain is engaged, according to advanced brain-image scans. When the elements of Medical Meditation are added, however, there is new activity in deeper anatomic structures of the brain, including the amygdala, other areas of the hippocampus, and the pons.

Following is a graph from that study, which clearly indicates the valuable effect of Medical Meditation upon the brain. In this case, the memory center of the brain, or hippocampus, receives a tremendous increase in activity following Medical Meditation.

Another example of the heightened power of Medical Meditation comes from a study by Shanti Shanti K. Khalsa, Ph.D. The study involved AIDS patients. Dr. Shanti Shanti tested Medical Meditation against mindfulness meditation, hoping to see which approach would better foster the quality of self-efficacy in AIDS patients. This quality—the perception of being able to adequately affect one's own environment—is pivotally

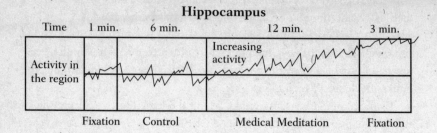

Hippocampus

| Time | 1 min. | 6 min. | 12 min. | 3 min. |

Activity in the region

Increasing activity

Fixation   Control   Medical Meditation   Fixation

important among AIDS patients, as well as to anyone else seeking to recover from illness. As Dr. Shanti Shanti indicated, self-efficacy enables AIDS patients to experience enhanced immune function, to have more satisfying social relationships, and to more fully engage in positive health behaviors. All three of these qualities are strong indicators of increased survival among AIDS patients. Dr. Shanti Shanti found that Medical Meditation had a more dynamic effect than mindfulness meditation, and more powerfully evoked self-efficacy.

These variations in effectiveness have prompted Harvard Medical School's Steele Belok, M.D., to remark that: "Some people may think that all meditative techniques are the same—that if you practice one procedure for reducing stress or developing your inner potential, you get the same results as you would from any other. But this has not held up under the scrutiny of research."

Current ongoing studies that may also corroborate the intrinsic advantage of the full-service approach of Medical Meditation include:

- A study at Beth Israel Deaconess Hospital affiliated with Harvard Medical School on the effects of Breath of Fire and segmented breathing, compared to the relaxation response, and a control period of normal breathing

- A study at Beth Israel Deaconess Hospital on the effects of Medical Meditation on heart rate; heart rate variability in response to stressors; muscle tension (measured by electromyelography); brain waves (measured by electroencephalography); and metabolic rate

- A proposed study at Harvard Medical School on the effects of Medical Meditation on the physiology of hormone release
- A proposed study at the University of Virginia School of Medicine, Department of Endocrinology, on the effects of Medical Meditation as an antiaging modality, focusing on its actions upon the hypothalamus and pituitary
- A proposed study at the University of Arizona jointly sponsored by the Departments of Psychology and Integrative Medicine in conjunction with the Alzheimer's Prevention Foundation, on the effects of Medical Meditation on memory function
- A study at California Pacific Medical Center, UCSF, in conjunction with the Guru Ram Das Center for Medicine and Humanology, on the effects of Medical Meditation done at a distance on diabetes.

Although these studies are not completed, I believe that the conclusions will confirm that Medical Meditation can play a powerful and positive role in the clinical setting.

PART TWO

The Healing Elements
of Medical Meditation

CHAPTER FOUR

Breath

The Kiss of God

You can fly. You can make love to a movie star. You can rule the world. In your dreams. But doing all these things is possible only if you know the technique called lucid dreaming—actively controlling your dreams, while still asleep. If you cannot do this—and most people don't know how—your dreams are far more likely to be mundane, with you as a passive observer.

Lucid dreaming is a cognitive condition that fascinates a number of researchers, including Stephen LaBerge, director of the Lucidity Institute, which is associated with Stanford University. LaBerge himself has been able to achieve as many as twenty-six lucid dreams per month, in which he has experienced his wildest fantasies. As he researched dreams, LaBerge punctured the old Freudian concept that dreams are messages from the subconscious, and that people are puppets of their unconscious urges. In fact, LaBerge showed in his research, dreams are "an improvised interaction between unconsciousness and consciousness." He further showed that this interaction can be carefully controlled.

The implication of this research is fascinating and profound. It means that the human psyche, with training, can voluntarily bounce between, and even merge, consciousness and unconsciousness. It means, in short, that we can control the supposedly uncontrollable.

Doing this, though, takes effort and exercise. One of the exercises that LaBerge does is to remember to ask himself, during a dream, Am I dreaming? LaBerge has found that the best way to remember to ask this question is to ask the same question while awake, many times each day. When people do this, LaBerge says, they frequently find that they are not dreaming but are not fully awake either—they are sleepwalking through their daily activities, only partly conscious of what they're doing. In this condition, their subconscious mind is often dominant, but not in a healthy way. It's often racing from one thought to another. Very frequently, these thoughts are fearful and anxious, because people, neurologically programmed for survival, are constantly looking for the next threat. Posing the question, Am I dreaming? however, snaps people out of their anxious daydreams and reawakens them to real life.

As part of this exercise, LaBerge and other lucid dreamers try to remember to touch the frame of every door through which they walk as they ask themselves, Am I dreaming? When they're not sleeping, this door-touching exercise wakes them up to life, by making them conscious of even such simple acts as walking through a door.

If you fear that you may be sleepwalking through much of your own life, try touching door frames. You'll find that it's quite difficult. You'll find that you're often just trudging through the motions of being alive, with little conscious awareness of what you're doing or where you are. Like many people, you will notice that you are often trapped in an anxious netherworld between consciousness and unconsciousness, worried about the future, regretful about the past, and oblivious to the only time that truly exists: the current moment.

The ancient yoga masters were also extremely concerned about the common human condition of sleepwalking through life. They devised their own system of overcoming it, a system that has endured for centuries, because it works on many levels. The system they devised for learning to control the uncontrollable, and to become conscious, was the control of breath.

The control of breath is the foundation of advanced meditation. It is the doorway to consciousness. That is why it is the first functional element of Medical Meditation that we will examine.

The Spirit of Breath

My colleague and fellow Tucson resident Andrew Weil, M.D., has noted that breathing is the only human act that people can do completely consciously or completely unconsciously, voluntarily or involuntarily. Because of this, breathing is controlled by two different sets of muscles and nerves, both of which can operate independently.

Most people, of course, breathe unconsciously almost all of the time. By doing this, they lose a tremendous opportunity—the chance to wake up, and become conscious of each moment. They also lose the chance to exercise their wills, and to take control of their most fundamental, constant human act. This loss of control can eventually lead to loss of control in other areas, until finally a person becomes powerless.

In addition, unconscious breathing is often quite ineffective, as are many other acts when they're done without purpose or control. It's estimated that approximately one-third of all people don't even breathe well enough to sustain normal health. These people don't get enough oxygen, don't eliminate enough carbon dioxide, don't sufficiently activate pulmonary neuropeptides, don't give the heart the support it needs, and don't adequately program the autonomic nervous system to operate in the healing, parasympathetic mode. This set of interrelated health insults causes innumerable problems. The most obvious are pulmonary problems, such as asthma and congestive lung disorders. However, because the body is comprised of a network of interlocking, interdependent systems, breathing problems can also cause cardiovascular disorders, mood disorders, immune deficiency, liver and digestive problems, and a wide variety of other pathologies.

These problems, though, are just the gross physical manifestations of improper breathing. The proper control of breath, as I mentioned, works on more than just one level. It also has a strong impact upon our ethereal level of being. When you breathe, you don't just breathe in a gaseous mixture containing oxygen. You also breathe in *prana*, the universal life force. The ancient yoga masters were far more interested in this ethereal aspect of breathing than in the obvious physical aspect—and rightly so, I believe.

The word *prana* is derived from the Sanskrit word meaning "absolute energy." Prana is the principal element, the vital force, that distinguishes living entities from inanimate objects. The sage Vivekananda eloquently defined prana as "a manifestation of the universal power, indefinite and omnipresent." According to the ancient masters, prana is the mystical force that is found in all living physical entities, but which is nonphysical. It is in air without being air. It is in water without being water. It is in food without being food. It can be experienced, or felt, but it cannot be seen, or heard.

The ancients said that wherever there is life in the universe, there is prana, and that without prana the universe would be dead, lifeless matter.

From a Western philosophical perspective, prana might be conceived of as the idea or spirit underlying matter. From a Western scientific perspective, prana has been conceived of as a form of radiation, of an indeterminate wavelength.

Animals, and particularly human beings, are believed to have a unique, almost magical relationship with prana, due to their capacity for cognition. The ancients believed man's cognitive ability endowed him with the power to receive, transfer, and transmit prana. This belief is similar to the more modern belief espoused by the Christian Science religion. In *Science and Health, with Keys to the Scriptures,* Christian Science founder Mary Baker Eddy wrote, "There exists a mutual influence between the celestial bodies, the earth, and animated things. Animal bodies are susceptible to the influence of this agent, disseminating itself through the substances of the nerves." The nerves that Eddy speaks of were conceived by the yoga masters as the *nadis,* the network of approximately 72,000 nonphysical energy conduits that carry prana throughout the body.

Prana is believed to enter the human body in many ways, but mostly through breathing. The reason for this is that breathing is our primary form of energy exchange with the environment. For example, we can go for weeks without food, and days without water, but only a few minutes without air. Breath is life, and life is but a series of breaths. From our first breath until our dying gasp, we inhale tremendous volumes of air. This air is a vast, diverse sample of our planet's entire atmosphere, which mixes at its outer extremities with space itself. In fact, a popular exercise for advanced mathematics students is to prove that each breath of air we breathe contains a molecule of the air from Jesus Christ's final breath on earth.

According to the tenets of kundalini yoga, as prana enters the body, it awakens human healing energy, or kundalini energy. The purpose of Kundalini Yoga exercises is to circulate this human prana, or kundalini energy, and to eventually return it to the cosmos. For this to efficiently occur, though, there must be sufficient replacement of prana, mostly from breathing.

Yoga masters are adept at inhaling enough air to provide abundant prana. They do this by using specific breathing techniques, which I'll soon show you. They are also adept at channeling, circulating, and even storing this pranic energy.

As I've noted, prana is in air, but it is not air. Therefore, it does not necessarily go to the lungs when inhaled, as air does. Yoga masters and advanced meditators have the rare ability to channel their incoming prana directly to the third-eye point. This produces a unique visual effect, a perception of a deep and luminous violet color. Meditators can then transfer this prana to their fifth chakra, near the thyroid, or to the heart chakra, or to any other region where energy is needed. This is primarily achieved through the Kundalini Yoga exercises and Medical Meditations that I am showing you in this book.

When it is time to return this kundalini energy to the universe, it can be channeled to the topmost crown chakra, or even released through the fingers. This energy, however, can also be retained in the body. Your body is capable of storing kundalini energy just as surely as a storage battery stores electricity. A person who has mastered the art of inhaling abundant amounts of prana, and activating it as kundalini energy, radiates great stored vitality.

Many of the masters of kundalini, including Westerners who do not use the language of yoga, are known as great healers. Well-conducted scientific testing has established that a rare few people have the power to frequently heal certain disorders with touch. With their hands, they can also affect inanimate fields of energy, such as magnetic fields, or noncognitive living things, such as plants.

The abilities of these people, however, are not always reliant upon physical forces, such as touch, because prana itself is not a physical force. Many of these people have notably heightened mental powers, such as intuition, and even a degree of telepathy and precognition. They also have an enhanced ability for distant healing—helping to heal others who are not directly present, through prayer and mental focus. I know that a concept such as distant healing may sound far-fetched to the uninitiated, but this phenomenon has been well documented in several recent studies by scientific pioneers in the field of spiritual healing, such as Larry Dossey, M.D., and Elisabeth Targ, M.D.

For rationalistic Westerners, some of the most impressive evidence of heightened pranic power comes from the observations of Eastern mystics. Some of these observations have become blurred and caricaturized in the recounting, to the point of being reduced to cartoonlike anecdotes of mystics lying on beds of nails, or walking over hot coals. Other observations, though, have been more accurately and vividly rendered, in books such as Yogananda's *Autobiography of a Yogi,* or Peter Kelder's *Ancient Secrets of the*

Fountain of Youth. Kelder, for example, writes of Alexandra David-Neel, a Frenchwoman who lived in Tibet and studied the secrets of the ancient masters. David-Neel, among other feats, was able to master the advanced yogi breathing technique known as *tumo,* which generates great heat. Using the tumo technique, she was able to travel in the icy Tibetan winters in light clothing. Monks that she met were able to actually melt the snow and ice around them, using tumo. In this chapter, I'll show you a variation of tumo, Breath of Fire, that you can master yourself.

Equally impressive feats of breath control—or *pranayama* in the Sanskrit—were reported in the 1946 book *Autobiography of a Yogi.* One account describes a yoga master performing the powerful bellows breathing exercise (which is similar to the Breath of Fire): "The master performed it before me with such amazing force that it seemed an actual storm had arisen in the room! Then he extinguished the thundering breath and remained motionless in a high state of superconsciousness. The aura of peace after the storm was vivid beyond forgetting."

In another episode, the author and a yoga master were sleeping outdoors when a swarm of mosquitoes descended. The attack was so fierce that the author became alarmed. He approached the master, who was not being bitten at all. It seemed as if the master were protected by a shield. The author found the master to be in a trance: "He was not breathing. His heart must have failed! I placed a mirror under his nose; no breath vapor appeared. To make doubly certain, for minutes I closed his mouth and nostrils with my fingers. His body was cold and motionless. In a daze, I turned toward the door to summon help.

"Then the master awoke, saying, 'So! A budding experimentalist! My poor nose!' The master's voice was shaky with laughter. 'Why don't you go to bed? Is the whole world going to change for you? Change yourself: Be rid of the mosquito consciousness.'"

A much more recent dramatic example of pranayama comes from the current free-diving champion of the world, Francisco Ferreras, who has had extraordinary control of his breath since childhood. Ferreras, who can dive one hundred feet underwater with no breathing apparatus, was born in Cuba, and was trained and studied by Soviet Union scientists. One feat that particularly impressed the scientists was Ferreras's ability to hold his breath for eight minutes, long past the point where most people would have died.

In the 1990s Ferreras visited Milan, Italy, and met a local yoga master. Ferreras demonstrated his extraordinary power of holding his breath to the yogi. The yogi decided to try it himself—and was timed at more than four-teen minutes on his first attempt. This amazing feat astonished Ferreras, who immediately began to study pranayama and meditation. Now Ferreras is an accomplished yogi himself. Ferreras credits pranayama and medita-tion with helping to further build his lung power. More significantly, it has increased his spiritual power, and given meaning to his efforts.

These few dramatic anecdotes are just a minute part of a much larger, almost universal regard for the spiritual importance of breathing. For exam-ple, the word *inspiration* literally means "to breathe in." In Sanskrit, the word *prana* means not only "universal life force," but also "breath." The Greek word for breath, *pneuma,* also means "soul," and "spirit." In Tibetan Buddhism, breath is referred to as the vehicle of the mind. In Hebrew, the word for breath also means "spirit of God." In Latin, *anima spiritus* means "breath" or "soul." The Japanese word for the universal energy (or prana), *ki,* also means "air."

Furthermore, in several different cultures, including those of Islam and India, it is believed that age is determined not so much by chronology as by the number of breaths a person takes. Each person is thought to be granted a specific number of breaths at birth. Thus, a person who breathes quickly will die sooner than a person who breathes slowly. In Indian yoga, there is an adage, "Breathlessness is deathlessness."

Going for long periods without breathing may sound unattainable for the average person, but it's not. This phenomenon is not uncommon dur-ing meditation. In fact, during the first scientific research on meditation, conducted at UCLA in the late 1960s, it was found that some meditators slowed their respiration to one breath per minute. Interestingly, the mental state that corresponded with the suspension of breath was a perception of complete awareness, or total knowledge.

In Asian cultures, it is also widely believed that the rhythm of breath is mankind's own signature vibration, which unites man with the vibratory force of the universe. Modern Asian yogis have stated that the vibration of human breath interlocks the finite magnetic field of humankind with the infinite magnetic field of the universe. The ebb and flow of breath is seen as a link to the motions and tides of the entire cosmos, outside our bodies, and within our bodies.

Because mankind is born of substance as well as spirit, though, there are also very practical, physical reasons for the importance of proper breathing. Let's consider them too, because they are integral to the fabric of your wholeness. I believe that proper breathing is indispensable to health and healing.

The Physiology of Breath

Every cell in the body is utterly dependent upon oxygen. Without oxygen, no cell can continue to live for more than a very limited number of minutes. Furthermore, if a cell is receiving just enough oxygen to stay alive, but not enough to thrive, its function declines markedly. When it happens to muscle tissue cells, they hurt. When it happens to brain cells, it causes a feeling of emotional distress. This is why certain obstructive lung diseases, such as emphysema, have a psychological component. Emphysema patients often suffer from mood disorders and a general feeling of malaise.

Conversely, though, if the cells of the body and brain are receiving an abundant supply of oxygen, this oxygen confers feelings of energy and optimal mood.

Oxygen enters the bloodstream in the lungs, through the alveolar sacs, and attaches to the hemoglobin of red blood cells, which carry it throughout the body. When a cell receives oxygen from a capillary, it exchanges an approximately equal amount of the gaseous waste carbon dioxide, which is carried back to the lungs and expelled through exhalation. This energy exchange occurs every moment of your life.

Inhalation occurs by contraction of the three diaphragm muscles, chiefly the large diaphragm muscle at the base of the lungs. When the diaphragm contracts, air pressure naturally fills the lungs. The contraction of the diaphragm, and the associated expansion of the lungs, exerts a number of critically important functions. One is the stimulation of blood circulation. As more oxygen is brought into the body, and absorbed by the alveoli, more blood must be pumped by the heart. This, of course, has a tremendously positive effect upon the body. Blood circulation is the prime physical nourisher of the body and brain, and the mechanism for cellular waste disposal.

Blood circulation is also enhanced by the effect of the lungs on the liver. The large vein that constantly supplies blood to the heart from the liver is partially emptied through mechanical suction developed by the lungs through breathing. When breathing is shallow or irregular, this action slows, and blood accumulates in the liver, causing swelling. This decreases blood flow in general, and especially decreases blood flow to the alimentary canal, the site of the body's digestive functions. When the alimentary canal doesn't get enough blood, it causes digestive problems.

In fact, poor digestion is one of the most common reactions to shallow breathing. I had one male patient who had been plagued by heartburn and gas for many years, but this condition gradually went away when he learned to breathe more slowly and deeply. Deep, slow breathing provides more blood to the alimentary canal, because the lungs literally suck up excess blood that has accumulated in the liver.

Because of the profound effect of breathing upon circulation, the diaphragm is sometimes referred to as the second heart.

Another effect of conscious breathing is the toning of the nervous system, including the peripheral nerves (which yogis believe are associated with the nadis). Pranayama that is especially effective for toning the nervous system includes rhythmic breathing exercises, such as the Breath of Fire.

Still another important physiological effect of proper breathing is the direct cleansing of the lungs. This is very important in our industrial society, because of the ubiquity of air pollution and airborne viruses, bacteria, and allergens. All of these toxins commonly enter the body through the lungs. It's impossible to ever completely empty the lungs of air, and various pollutants, because of the lungs' spongy construction. However, deep, powerful breaths do eliminate a great deal of toxic and noxious debris. In my practice, I have seen patients recover quickly from respiratory infections when they did breathing exercises. I also am convinced that conscious breathing can prevent respiratory infections, including the common cold. Breathing exercises also appear to confer a high degree of immunity to tuberculosis (which appears to be increasing in incidence). This was recently proven in research conducted at the Yoga Research Institute in Longwala, India.

Another extremely important physical aspect of breathing is its effect upon mood. As I'm sure you've noticed, one of the best ways to calm yourself, and escape either fear or anger, is to breathe deeply. Deep breathing is also excellent at reducing pain, as women who have used Lamaze deep breathing during childbirth know.

One important reason breathing affects mood and pain is because of its impact upon a part of the brain known as the periaqueductal gray area, or PAG. The PAG, located in the aqueduct that connects the third and fourth ventricles in the midbrain, is an important nodal point, where many nerves come together. Of special importance, this nodal point is the site of the body's largest supply of opiate receptors. Therefore, the PAG is instrumental in determining a person's pain threshold. The PAG also helps to control anger and fear, since the body's opiates can help decrease these uncomfortable emotional feelings.

The lungs have a direct effect upon the PAG. As you may recall, the lungs are filled with a very high concentration of peptides, the partial proteins that are involved in thought and feeling. Therefore, the lungs have their own form of intelligence, and can communicate with the brain's PAG via these peptides (which are released into the cerebrospinal fluid).

Pranayama, or breath control, changes the type and amount of peptides that reach the PAG. By breathing deeply, or rapidly, or by holding your breath, you can change your profile of pulmonary peptides, and communicate with your brain's periaqueductal gray area. This changes how you feel. You can use this mechanism to reduce pain, anger, or fear.

This relief from pain, anger, and fear is not only satisfying in and of itself but also a powerful spur to healing. New research has shown consistent, powerful, positive shifts in mood when the correct type of breathing is used in a walking meditation program. Moreover, energy levels are rapidly elevated while chronic pain is diminished. Healing occurs in the sacred space of calmness and confidence, not amid the turmoil of fear, anger, and pain. As Dr. Candace Pert has written, "This peptide substrate may provide the scientific rationale for the powerful healing effects of consciously controlled breath patterns."

Another reason that deep, controlled, rhythmic breathing helps heal is because it shifts the body away from the fight-or-flight mode. As I mentioned, breathing is the only action in the body that has a dual control system—it can operate consciously, through the voluntary nervous system, or unconsciously, through the autonomic nervous system. Because of this unique aspect, breathing is the one function of the body that can allow the voluntary nervous system to reprogram the autonomic nervous system.

This reprogramming can be an absolute godsend. The autonomic nervous system is your body's primary neurological defense against illness, but it often gets out of balance. Instead of operating in the healing, rest-and-repair parasympathetic mode, which favors the glands and organs of the immune system, it often operates far too much in the sympathetic, fight-or-flight mode. This generally happens because of stress that is not balanced by relaxation techniques, such as meditation. When this does happen, it pulls energy away from your immune system, and away from your various recovery mechanisms, and shifts this energy to the fight-or-flight organs: the muscles, the heart, the eyes, and so on.

When this happens too frequently for too long, it destroys the body. Opportunistic illnesses strike. Viruses spread. Bacteria proliferate. The glands and organs of the fight-or-flight mode become exhausted. The heart may begin to beat erratically. The endocrine glands that provide zest and youth degenerate. Muscles may begin to ache with symptoms of fibromyalgia. Chronic fatigue symptoms may appear. Aging sets in. Illness occurs.

This dire state, though, can be overcome with proper breathing. In a recent lecture, Dr. Andrew Weil described how simple breathing exercises enabled many of his patients to recover from conditions such as irregular heartbeat, atrial fibrillation, high blood pressure, and panic attacks. I, too, have had great success in helping patients recover from these types of conditions, using Medical Meditation, which almost always includes a breathing component.

As you can see, conscious breathing has three primary effects: (1) it heightens a person's overall consciousness, by prompting him or her to exert conscious control over a normally unconscious act; (2) it increases the amount of prana that enters the body; and (3) it has powerful physiological healing effects.

You can use your newfound expertise in breathing to gain greater effectiveness and enjoyment even in very simple things in life. For example, to increase your mindfulness of the moment, before you rise from sitting in a chair, inhale deeply through your nose, then stand up. This will increase your awareness. When you walk into a room full of people and have to say something or announce yourself, inhale, exhale, inhale again, and begin your presentation or your announcement. This can also work at parties, or other gatherings. Your newfound breath awareness will also help in your athletic activities, and even in your more intimate moments.

Whenever you get a chance, stop, inhale deeply, bring the energy up, and then exhale again through the nose. This will keep you calm, centered, relaxed, and at peace.

Now let's see what you can do to improve your own breathing. The following exercises can be done by themselves, and are also often incorporated into the Medical Meditations that I'll soon teach you. Try them. If you apply yourself, they will soon begin to change your life, and bring you more personal power and healing power than you thought possible.

Pranayama

The most important thing about breathing is to know how *not* to breathe. Unfortunately, this is probably how you now often breathe. Very few people breathe entirely correctly, and approximately one-third of all people breathe so poorly that it contributes to their ill health and lack of vitality.

The main problem most people have is that their breath is too shallow. The primary reason for this is physical tension, caused by stress. Unfortunately, this shallow breathing, or top-breathing, tends to further lock in tension and stress, creating a vicious cycle. A shallow breath fills only the top part of the lungs. It may cause the chest to expand, but that's not enough. The abdomen must expand too. The second most common reason for shallow breathing is bad posture. Many people slump so badly that it restricts their breathing. Other common reasons are tight clothing, being overweight, and smoking.

Following is the technique for proper breathing. I call this the Complete Breath. It's also sometimes called the Yogi Breath. You should inhale a series of Complete Breaths at least several times each day, trying to do this as frequently as possible. At first, this may be hard to remember to do, because you may be accustomed to breathing unconsciously. But now it's time to change your consciousness. It's time to stop sleepwalking and to change your life into exactly the life you want it to be. It's time to heal. Start with breathing. Everything starts with breathing.

Basic Breathing Exercises
THE COMPLETE BREATH

1. Stand or sit erect, with a straight spine.
2. Inhale steadily through the nostrils, filling the lower part of your lungs first. Your abdomen will push out.
3. Fill the middle part of the lungs, pushing out the lower ribs, breastbone and chest.
4. Fill the next highest part of the lungs, expanding and lifting the upper chest, and the upper six or seven pairs of ribs.
5. Draw the abdomen in slightly, to fill the highest part of the lungs.
6. Retain the breath for several seconds. This will allow maximum

contact with the alveolar surfaces, and result in optimal intake of oxygen.

7. Exhale quite slowly, holding the chest in a firm position, drawing the abdomen slightly inward and upward. When the air is completely exhaled, relax the chest and abdomen.

The Complete Breath should be taken in one smooth, continuous motion, and should take about 2 seconds to inhale, and somewhat longer to exhale. With practice, inhalation can be extended to 5–10 seconds. It may help to practice the Complete Breath in front of a mirror, with your hands on your abdomen, to feel the movements. Once you have learned this technique, you will find it innately pleasurable, and will tend to keep doing it. The Complete Breath is of vital importance to everyone. Children, though, and especially babies, usually breathe this way naturally.

The effects of the Complete Breath are:

- Increased calmness
- Reduction of toxins
- Increase in pranic intake
- Reduction of physical tension
- Enhanced oxygenation of the blood
- Increased consciousness of unconscious acts
- Synchronization of personal breath rhythm with universal vibration

Now let's look at some variations on the Complete Breath. These breathing exercises have powerful effects, and will be the cornerstones of your Medical Meditations.

YOGI NERVE REVITALIZING BREATH

This is an exercise practiced by virtually all yogis, who generally consider it one of the strongest nerve stimulants. It stimulates the central and peripheral nervous systems, and develops nerve force, energy, and vitality. It also brings stimulating pressure on several important nerve plexi that are associated with various chakras, which stimulates the entire nervous system and sends increased peripheral nerve force to all parts of the body.

1. Stand erect, inhale a Complete Breath, and retain it.
2. Extend your arms in front of you loosely, in a relaxed way.

3. Slowly move your hands back to your shoulders, as you squeeze your fists increasingly hard.
4. With your fists clenched very tightly, push them out and draw them back rapidly, several times.
5. Exhale vigorously through the mouth.

The effects of the Yogi Revitalizing Breath are:

- Increased circulation
- Toning of nerve function
- Release of epinephrine and norepinephrine
- Movement of kundalini to higher chakras

THE RETAINED BREATH

This form of pranayama strengthens the muscles of the lung and expands the chest. It also increases oxygenation of the blood, which is of particular benefit to the liver and the other organs of digestion. In addition, it enhances the exit of blood-borne toxins through the lungs.

When you do this exercise, do not hold the breath longer than 10 seconds, because this can sometimes cause dizziness. As Yogi Bhajan has noted, dizziness is not enlightenment.

1. Standing or sitting erect, inhale a Complete Breath through your nose, pulling in your chin.
2. Retain the air for 10 seconds, as you remain still and calm. If you have the urge to exhale, inhale slightly instead.
3. Exhale through the nose.

Throughout this exercise, create a calm internal spot in your awareness, and observe the changes in your body and mind. Breath retention will make your body work at a higher level of efficiency. It will also train you to remain rational during stress or pressure. To master this is to master the inflow and outflow of the life force.

The effects of the Retained Breath are:

- Toning of chest muscles
- Heightened oxygenation
- Improved digestion and liver function
- Improved conscious awareness of breath
- Increased detoxification through the lungs

THE ONE-MINUTE BREATH

A variation of the Retained Breath is the One-Minute Breath, in which you take only one breath during one minute. Most people will find this difficult at first, and should work up to it by taking three breaths per minute, and then three breaths over two minutes. As a rule, people usually take about twelve to fourteen breaths per minute.

The one-minute breath is sometimes called the one-minute cure, because of its unique ability to change a negative thought, feeling, or vibration into a positive one. This is often the key to healing, because negativity has a notably deleterious physical effect. As your awareness increases, and you realize you have negativity in your mind, immediately go into the mechanics of the one-minute breath.

1. Inhale very gradually for 20 seconds through the nose.
2. Hold your breath in for 20 seconds, as you focus on the third-eye point, at the topmost root of the nose.
3. Exhale gradually for 20 seconds through your nose.
4. Then repeat.

If this proves to be too difficult, then begin by inhaling for 10 seconds through the nose, hold the breath for 10 seconds, and exhale through the nose for 10 seconds. With practice gradually increase this to 20 seconds each.

The effects of the One-Minute Breath are:

- Accelerated healing
- Increased flow of prana
- Heightened sexual energy
- An increase in cognitive energy
- An increase in creativity and intuition
- Increased blood circulation to the brain
- Increased calmness and sense of peace

THE BREATH WALK

Breath Walk is adapted from the work of my colleague Gurucharan Singh Khalsa, Ph.D., who is the author of the book *BreathWalk* and a related series of audiotapes. For information on the audiotapes, see Resources and Referrals.

In this exercise, you link your breath to the rhythm of your steps. This conscious linkage engages the mind, especially if you use a mantra to help connect your breaths and steps. This exercise is relaxing and energizing at the same time.

1. Walk with your head up, your chin drawn in slightly, and your shoulders back.
2. Inhale a Complete Breath, and count silently to four, taking a step with each count. Or repeat the four-syllable mantra, "Sa Ta Na Ma," silently.
3. Exhale slowly through the nostrils, with a count of four breaths and steps, or repeat the mantra.

From time to time, relax your breath patterns and walk normally. Be mindful of your surroundings.

There are variations to this technique. One is to add the mantra "Wahe Guru," on four counts, as you exhale. The mantra "Sa Ta Na Ma" will produce enhanced cognition and intuition, while "Wahe Guru" will help bring you to a state of ecstasy.

The effects of the Breath Walk are:

- Relaxation
- Energy increase
- Enhanced flow of prana
- Boost of blood circulation
- A conscious linkage between your own rhythm and that of the universe

RHYTHMIC BREATHING

Rhythmic Breathing is a form of breathing that places special emphasis on rhythm, or vibration. Rhythmic Breathing is of inestimable value in uniting a human being with the cosmos, because, from the tiniest atom to the greatest star, every entity in the universe is pulsing with vibration. In all of nature, there is nothing at absolute rest, not even a rock. In fact, some physicists believe that a single atom at rest would destroy the entire universe.

One elemental cause of vibration is change. Everything that exists, from inanimate objects to human beings, is in a state of change—either growth, decay, or mechanical transformation. Everything that has ever existed began to change the moment it was created. Matter is constantly being played upon by energy, and as this occurs, it creates a vibration, or rhythm. Certainly, the atoms in your body are in constant vibration, composing and decomposing your human form, and then returning to the universe. Scarcely a single atom that is now in your body was present in you a few months ago. As every moment has passed, you have been continually reborn. However, throughout this change, the unique vibrations that make you you, lodged deep in your own DNA, are ceaseless. These vibrations leave your body, enter the universe, and one day return. As astronomer Sir Arthur Eddington has said, "When the electron vibrates, the universe shakes."

Rhythmic Breathing helps unite your own vibrations with the eternal rhythm of the cosmos. It helps to capture cosmic vibration, and to implant it in your own vibration. This greatly increases the power of your vibration.

The effects of Rhythmic Breathing are somewhat analogous to the power that is generated when a number of people cross a bridge. If these people are marching rhythmically, it can create vibrations that are so strong they can destroy the bridge. For this reason, a column of soldiers always breaks step when crossing a bridge. In your own life, though, you want to tune in to the great rhythmic march of the universe, and thus tap its power.

1. Sit erect in a comfortable position, with your chest, neck, and head vertically aligned. Place your hands on your lap, and hold your shoulders slightly back.
2. Inhale a Complete Breath during 6 beats of your heart. (Take your pulse before beginning the exercise, to get a feel for the length of 6 heartbeats.)
3. Retain the breath for 3 heartbeats, and exhale it during 6 heartbeats.
4. Pause for 3 heartbeats between breaths.

Some yogis use Rhythmic Breathing as a meditation for healing, and also for blocking pain. To do this, they place their hands on the afflicted area, breathe rhythmically, and focus on the mental image of bringing prana to the affected area.

The effects of Rhythmic Breathing are:

• Relaxation
• Increased intake of oxygen

- Increased intake of prana
- Toning of the nervous system
- The connection of possibly disparate rhythms within the body, such as those of heartbeat and breath

THE BREATH OF FIRE ("AGNI PRAN")

This is a form of Rhythmic Breathing unique to kundalini yoga that creates energy. A rapid, powerful, diaphragmatic breath, it is an excellent tonic any time your energy begins to flag. Sometimes Breath of Fire will cause mild perspiration on the forehead. Yogis believe this is caused by *tapa,* or psychic energy. I like to call this breath the spark that kindles the flame.

The Breath of Fire may cause a slight feeling of lightheadedness, but does not create hyperventilation. Studies have shown that the Breath of Fire actually increases oxygen in the blood, while carbon dioxide levels remain stable.

Although you should begin to practice this for durations of 1 to 3 minutes, some people find it easy to do a full 10 minutes immediately. Some tingling sensations and lightheadedness are completely normal, as your body adjusts to the new stimulation of your nerves. If you concentrate at the brow point, this should pass quickly. Once you have adjusted, it normally stays away. In some people, this is the result of toxins released by the breath. That type of sensation is helped by a light diet, with a lot of fresh vegetable juices. Others find the breath creates initial dizziness or giddiness. These are signs you are not doing it correctly. Stop, rest, and then begin again.

To perform Breath of Fire:

1. Inhale through your nostrils by bringing your diaphragm down, instead of up. Breathe from your diaphragm, with your chest relaxed. Focus your mental energy on your third chakra, or solar plexus, which is the seat of your personal power.
2. Make your inhalations swift and powerful, more than one inhalation per second.
3. Do not pause between inhaling and exhaling.
4. Exhale forcefully through your nose.
5. Continue this for 1–3 minutes.

A variation: Sit straight and place your hands together in a prayer pose at the center of the chest. The fingers point upward and the thumbs press against the sternum. Close the eyelids nine-tenths of the way. Roll the eyes up and concentrate at the brow point. Begin Breath of Fire. Continue for 3 minutes, then inhale through the nose and hold for 10 seconds. Relax. Do Breath of Fire again, through the nose. Inhale through the nose and hold for 10 seconds, then exhale through the nose, and relax. Stay still and place the hands on the knees with the first fingertip touching the thumb, palms up. Watch the natural flow of the breath and the constant stream of sensation, both internal and external. After 3 minutes inhale deeply, and exhale. Repeat this combination of 3 minutes of Breath of Fire with 3 minutes of breath awareness for three to five repetitions.

The effects of the Breath of Fire are:

- Increase in endurance
- Increase of resistance to stress
- Reduction of addictive impulses
- Release of toxins from the mucous membranes of the lungs
- Enhanced balance of the sympathetic and parasympathetic nervous systems
- Stimulation of the splanchnic nerves, causing increased output of epinephrine and norepinephrine

Medical Meditation Breathing Exercises

BREATH AWARENESS EXERCISE

Tune in and center yourself by chanting "Ong Namo, Guru Dev Namo" 3 times (Tune on page 143).

Posture: Sit in Easy Pose or in a chair with your spine straight.

Focus: With your eyes closed, let all of your attention gather on your breath.

Breath: Breathe long, slow, and deep through the nose. Sense the breath as a quality of motion. How does it move in the different parts of your body as you breathe in a steady and meditative rhythm? What elements seem to dominate the quality of your own breath as you begin the exercise? How does that change as you continue to meditate?

Mantra: Mentally repeat "Sat" on the inhale, "Nam" on the exhale.

Meaning of mantra: "My true identity."

Mudra: The hands are in gyan mudra, with the index finger touching the thumb. (See page 95.)

Time: 3–11 minutes.

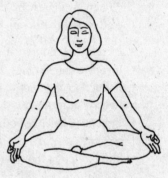

End: Inhale deeply through your nose and hold your breath for 10 seconds. Exhale through the nose. Repeat two more times, and relax.

COMMENTS: Feel the motion and live energy of the breath. Visualize the body as luminous. As you inhale, the light increases in brightness, extent, and penetration. Let that breath and light merge with the entire cosmos. Let the breath breathe you. Experience yourself as a unit and the cosmos as unlimited. Feel that you are a part of that vastness. The breath is a wave on an ocean of energy, of which you are a part.

The character of your thoughts and emotions is reflected in the motion and level of energy in your breath. One of the first habits of a yogi is to notice the state of the breath and prana. A disturbance in the prana foreshadows what will manifest in the body and emotions.

Yogi Bhajan has his students meditate in this manner for many hours. Practice this meditation with silence, and assess your energy state.

BASIC BREATH SERIES

Tune in and center yourself by chanting "Ong Namo, Guru Dev Namo" 3 times (Tune on page 143).

Posture: Sit in Easy Pose or in a chair with your spine straight.

Focus: The eyes are closed and focused at the third-eye point.

1. Breath: Raise your right hand in front of you to the right of the face, palm flat and facing left. The fingers are together and point straight up. Press the side of your thumb on the right nostril to gently close it. Begin long, slow, deep, complete yogic breaths through the left nostril. Inhale and exhale through the left nostril.

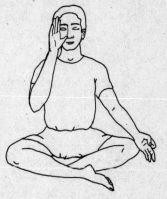

Mantra: Mentally repeat "Sat" on the inhale, "Nam" on the exhale.

Meaning of mantra: "My true identity."

Mudra: Rest your left hand on your left knee in gyan mudra, with the index finger touching the thumb. Your left arm is straight.

Time: 3 minutes.

End: Inhale; hold your breath for 10–30 seconds. Exhale.

2. Breath: Raise your left hand in front of and to the left of your face, palm flat, facing to the right. The fingers of the hand are together and point straight up. Press the side of your thumb on the left nostril to gently close it. Begin long, slow, deep, complete yogic breaths through the right nostril. Inhale and exhale through the right nostril.

Mantra: Mentally repeat "Sat" on the inhale, "Nam" on the exhale.

Meaning of mantra: "My true identity."

Mudra: Rest your right hand on your right knee in gyan mudra, with your index finger touching your thumb. Your right arm is straight.

Time: 3 minutes.

End: Inhale; hold your breath for 10–30 seconds. Exhale.

3. Breath: Raise your right hand in front of, and to the right of, your face, as in number 1. The palm is flat and faces to the left. Block your right nostril with your thumb. Press just hard enough to close the nostril. Keep the rest of your fingers

straight up. Inhale deeply through the left nostril. When the breath is full, bend your right hand into a "U" as you extend the little fingertip over, and press on your left nostril. Close your left nostril and let your right nostril open by releasing the thumb pressure. Exhale smoothly and completely through your right nostril. When the breath is completely exhaled, begin the cycle again with the inhale through your left nostril.

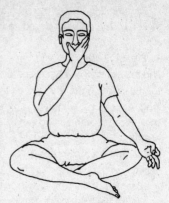

Mantra: Mentally repeat "Sat" on the inhale, "Nam" on the exhale.

Meaning of mantra: "My true identity."

Mudra: Rest your left hand on your left knee in gyan mudra, with your index finger touching your thumb. Your left arm is straight.

Time: 3 minutes.

End: Inhale; hold your breath for 10–30 seconds. Exhale.

4. Breath: Repeat the above exercise (number 3), except use your left hand to direct the inhale through your right nostril and exhale through your left nostril.

Mantra: Mentally repeat "Sat" on the inhale, "Nam" on the exhale.

Meaning of mantra: "My true identity."

Mudra: Rest your right hand on your right knee in gyan mudra, with your index finger touching your thumb. Your right arm is straight.

Time: 3 minutes.

End: Inhale; hold your breath for 10–30 seconds. Exhale.

5. Breath: Begin Breath of Fire. Keep the breath powerful, regular, and conscious.

Mantra: Mentally repeat "Sat" on the inhale, "Nam" on the exhale.

Meaning of mantra: "My true identity."

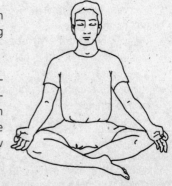

Mudra: Relax your hands on your knees in gyan mudra, with your index fingers touching your thumbs.

Time: 3 minutes.

End: Inhale and hold the breath for 10 seconds. Exhale. Mentally watch the energy circulate throughout the entire body. Relax the breath and concentrate on the natural flow of the breath as life force, for 3 minutes. Notice now how your mind and emotions have changed.

6. In the same posture, chant long "Sat Nam."
   Breath: The breath will come automatically as you chant.
   Mantra: "Sat Nam."
   Meaning of mantra: "My true identity."
   Mudra: Hands are in gyan mudra, with your index fingers touching your thumbs, and are relaxed on your knees.
   Time: 3–11 minutes.
   End: Inhale; hold your breath for 10–30 seconds. Exhale.

COMMENTS: This set gives you a quick lift in energy, increased clarity, and a sense of balance. If you do the minimum time for each exercise, it only takes 22–25 minutes to completely reset yourself. It is an excellent set for beginners. You learn your relationship to your breath, and you observe the differences in emotion and thinking that each type of breathing creates.

Even though breathing is the most natural and essential thing we do, conscious breathing can be quite a challenge. When you alter the breath, you begin to oppose and release the habitual patterns of emotion and attention that are coded in the habits of your body and mind. As those patterns begin to alter, you may drift in concentration. However, if you continue, and command the breath, then you will gain a new sense of control.

THE 4/4 BREATH FOR ENERGY

Tune in and center yourself by chanting "Ong Namo, Guru Dev Namo" 3 times (tune on page 143).
   Posture: Sit in Easy Pose or in a chair with your spine straight.
   Focus: The eyes are closed and focused at the third-eye point.
   Breath: All breathing is done through the nose. Inhaling, break the breath into 4 equal parts or sniffs, filling the lungs completely on the 4th. As you exhale, release the breath equally in 4 parts, completely emptying the lungs on the 4th. On each part of the inhale and exhale, pull in your navel point. The stronger you pump the navel point, the more energy you will generate. One full breath cycle (in and out) takes about 7–8 seconds.

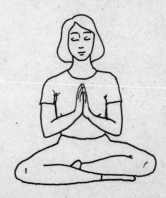

   Mantra: "Sa Ta Na Ma," to be repeated mentally on both the inhale and the exhale.
   Meaning of mantra: This mantra represents the cycle of creation. Sa means infinity; Ta means life; Na means death; Ma means rebirth.
   Mudra: Bring your hands into prayer pose at the center of your chest. The palms are together and your fingers are pointing up.

Time: 2–3 minutes.

End: Inhale, hold the breath, and press the palms forcefully together for 10 seconds, creating a tension in the whole body. Hold as long as possible. Exhale. Repeat the inhale, hold, exhale cycle two more times and feel all the tension in your body vanish.

COMMENTS: If you press the hands together very hard, and do this Medical Meditation vigorously, 1 minute will recharge you and alter your mental state.

This will relax and energize you, and help combat encroaching fatigue or negative emotion. This is a great, quick pickup when you have only a minute. If you do it 2 or 3 times a day at strategic times, you will notice a big difference in the way you feel.

Although this breathing technique may seem similar to Breath of Fire, it is quite different. The former is a rapid, diaphragmatic, quick and shallow breath, while this is a long, deep breath divided into 4 segments. With a little practice you can easily master this technique.

Breath is your primary source of energy, both physical and ethereal. Everything starts with breath. To use the energy that breath brings, though, you must master the control of your postures and movements. Posture and movement control the flow of physical energy and ethereal energy within the body.

Therefore, let us continue our journey into healing by analyzing the power of movement. Without the controlling power of movement, energy will still exist, but will be merely a chaotic whirlwind. With proper control of movement, you can forge your energy into a healing force.

CHAPTER FIVE

Posture and Movement

Why Was I Born into This Body?

My patient, Alesandra, was a tangle of awkward angles. Her body was graced by neither balance nor flexibility. Her arms and legs moved so mechanically that she looked almost like a marionette. As Alesandra teetered uncomfortably on her chair—her face an immobile mask, her movements robotic—she told me that she wanted to find a way to mentally escape from her body, which was causing her great torment because of chronic pain. She'd read an article about my work with Medical Meditation, and seemed to consider it a means of escape. She was right to think that Medical Meditation might help, but she didn't understand its mechanism of action. Medical Meditation wouldn't divorce her from her body; instead it would unite her with it, and give her a chance to heal it.

Alesandra, forty-one, had an excruciating, often fatal autoimmune disorder called polymyositis. Her own body had turned against itself, and was setting her muscles on fire with inflammation. She was trying to be brave, but the harder she tried, the more her pain showed. Her stoicism was just a posture, and it didn't fit. Every time she squared her shoulders and set her chin, her face went white, and the symmetry of her body collapsed.

She was taking steroids to depress her immunity and reduce her autoimmune response, but the drugs had created acne that was so severe she couldn't even touch her own face without irritating the sores on it. Her primary care physician had told her that in a relatively short time she would be confined to a wheelchair, and would then probably contract pneumonia and die.

At one point during our consultation, she made the mistake of scratching her cheek, and the moment she did it, she jerked her hand away, shuddered in pain, and gasped. As she caught her breath, she looked at the floor and moaned, "Why me?" Then she looked me in the eye. "Why was I born into this body?"

I could have told her, I suppose, that we're all born into bodies that betray us, bodies that begin as vulnerable and weak, that blossom ever so briefly, and then begin to decline even in our early twenties, until before we know it, we're weak once more. But she wasn't ready to hear that. She felt so isolated by her pain—as do most chronic pain patients—that she considered herself set apart, singled out for special punishment. I'd once had another polymyositis patient, Scott, and he'd felt exactly the same way: "Why me?"

So instead I simply said, "That's an excellent question. Why you? I can't tell you why, myself. But I think you can find the answer. And when you do, it's going to do more than anything else to ease your suffering. Did you ever hear of Victor Frankl, the psychiatrist who was in a Nazi concentration camp? He said that people can endure almost anything, as long as they can find meaning in it. He did a study of concentration camp survivors and found that the one thing they most had in common wasn't youth or strength, but the ability to find meaning in their suffering."

She looked bewildered. "How on earth do I find a meaning in this—if there is a meaning?"

I told her about the best soul-searching method I know: Medical Meditation. I thought it was her best therapeutic option—maybe her only viable option. The drugs she was taking held no hope of a cure, and weren't even adequately controlling her symptoms. But I had seen Medical Meditation work wonders against mysterious, arcane diseases like hers. It had helped my patient Scott immensely.

Hopefully, Medical Meditation would bring her closer to her highest self, the part of her that is not in pain, nor even frightened about death. Many of my chronic pain patients have successfully found a way to contact their highest selves, because they have the strongest possible motivation a person can have: escape from torture. The terrible threat of pain has empowered many of these people to achieve things that most healthy people can't imagine. Many of my pain patients have learned to control their broken bodies like yogis, and to be masters of their own perceptions. Simply put, they have learned to reinterpret their pain signals. This may sound impossibly difficult, but it's really not. Even a relatively simple medication such as nitrous oxide—the laughing gas that dentists use—enables ordinary people to actually experience pain sensations, but to neurologically interpret them in a new, nonthreatening way. Yogis and advanced meditators have a similar ability, without drugs.

I also hoped, though, that Medical Meditation might help Alesandra in another very important way. I hoped it would help end her pain, by reconditioning and reprogramming her nervous system.

Some of Alesandra's pain was likely caused by the ongoing inflammation of her acute illness; as with most chronic pain patients, Alesandra suffered from engraved pain—pain that literally becomes programmed into the anatomy of the nervous system. Pain becomes engraved upon the nervous system when the gates in the spinal cord that help protect people from pain are bombarded by repeated, chronic pain signals, millions of times per hour. This ceaseless assault jams open the gates of pain and creates a neurological pathway that requires no further stimulus. The pain literally develops a life of its own, and a person can continue to hurt even after an injury or illness has healed. For example, if a leg is in great pain because of an injury, or because of cancer, the patient can continue to experience this pain even after the leg is amputated. This phantom limb pain, which is quite common, is the result of overstimulated nerve pathways.

I was hopeful that much of Alesandra's physical change would come from the kundalini yoga elements of Medical Meditation. The postures, movements, and hand positions of kundalini yoga have a startling power over the physical condition of the body. Yoga, as a stand-alone therapy, has helped millions of people to achieve astonishing physical feats. As you may recall, recent medical research has proven that yoga alone can be a powerful medical modality for many diseases.

Of course, yoga virtually always includes breath control, which is itself a singular force for restoring health. In addition, Medical Meditation also adds the elements of mental focus and mantra, which bring the power of yoga to a whole new level. When the postures, the breath exercises, the movements, the hand positions, the mental focus, and the mantras of Medical Meditation are all performed together, in the proper sequence, the resulting exercise is called a *kriya*. Because kriyas consist of numerous, interlocking, synergistic elements, they are immeasurably more powerful than just isolated yoga postures and movements.

In this chapter, I will tell you how to achieve therapeutic intervention with postures, movements, and hand positions, used in various combinations as kriyas. These elements are a major part of Medical Meditation.

From Self-Consciousness to the Conscious Self

When an Olympic marathoner wins a gold medal, it's not the piece of gold he or she remembers always—it's the race. It is the pain, and the victory over pain, that graces the rest of the runner's life. It is the intense, absolute involvement with the running of that race that forever gives meaning to the runner's existence.

Most spectators consider running to be a simple sport—putting one foot in front of the other—but the act is very complex for those who do it at the highest level. It demands focus. Great runners must telescope the entire force of their mind, body, and spirit into every moment of foot torsion, upper body synchronization, and linkage of breath to movement. They must bring an otherworldly consciousness to this one natural act.

The same intensity of focus and attention to detail is necessary for meditators who are trying to defeat deadly illnesses. I often tell my gravely ill patients that they must be willing to train as hard as Olympic athletes. Many of them do, and achieve the same reward as world-class athletes: a sense of peace and power that is quite extraordinary.

Much of what creates a great athlete, as well as a great meditator, is the ability to become acutely conscious of the simple actions that most people perform unconsciously. In Medical Meditation, these actions include not just breathing, but also postures and movements. Advanced meditators are just as conscious of their movements and postures as they are of their breathing and their state of mind. In fact, the Sanskrit word for yoga postures, *asanas,* means to be present.

Yogi Bhajan has noted that when meditators assume yoga postures, it makes them conscious of particular areas of their bodies. As they hold these postures, which sometimes requires work, they become uncomfortably self-conscious about the effort. When meditators rigorously apply themselves, though, this self-consciousness leads to the much more enlightening condition of being conscious about oneself. With even more effort, this consciousness about oneself can allow a person to be, as Yogi Bhajan says, "a conscious self."

As a person struggles to become a conscious self, wondrous things occur. As a rule, when most people initially begin to assume the postures of yoga, their most fundamental posture, in the larger sense of the word, is that of the ego. We all tend to posture, or pose, as self-confident, powerful people, even though we may feel weak and afraid inside. The postures of yoga, though, help us to find the true power that lies within. This happens for several reasons. One is that the postures of yoga frequently require discipline, and the exercise of discipline builds power. More importantly, though, the postures of yoga help awaken and channel the internal energy, or kundalini, that lies coiled inside us, and it is this kundalini energy that is the ultimate source of our true personal power. With it, we can perform almost supernatural feats, and can attain the sense of independence and serenity that is common among yogis.

When people achieve this independence and serenity, they invariably make a personal commitment to themselves to retain this amazing, new-found power. This commitment to keep up their power changes the way that they project themselves to the outer world. As Yogi Bhajan puts it, "They start to look like infinity. That's what yoga posture is all about. It's very practical. There's no philosophy in yoga that doesn't come with some way of engaging the body, to give you that experience. There's no such thing as an abstract concept, without a posture or sadhana to give you the capacity to experience it."

The postures of kundalini yoga, as well as other forms of yoga, are intended to coax the body out of old ways of holding itself, and moving. Often these old ways are rigid and imbalanced. They were created as a defensive posture against stress, fear, and pain. They may have worked well for a short time in the past, but over the long course of a lifetime, they are a deadly trap. They sap the body of energy, and cause pain of their own. Muscles can literally be cemented, with connective tissue, to tendons, ligaments, and other muscles. When this occurs, stress can be locked into the body. Many bodywork therapists have found that when deep tissues are therapeutically relaxed, it often triggers a release of emotion. This may be due in part to the neurological chemicals that are present throughout the body, in our various nodal-point hot spots.

When the body's posture is out of alignment, it also frequently causes people to move awkwardly. It's impossible to be graceful or physically efficient when one's back, neck, arms, and legs are hobbled with stiffness and tension. Just as poor posture assaults physical vitality, so does stiff, inefficient movement. Yoga postures and movements, however, help to correct poor posture and inefficient movements. They break up old ways of standing, sitting, walking, and working, and replace them with more graceful ones.

As this happens, it fundamentally changes people. In the larger sense, it enables people to become aware of and to break away from other stratified aspects of their lives, such as unhealthy attachments, habits, and relationships. It even helps them to transform their two deepest, most innate relationships: that between now and forever, and that between their individual self and the universal self.

On a very practical level, yoga postures and movements also help people to achieve two of the most vitally important aspects of healing: flexibility and balance.

Flexibility

Flexibility is of paramount importance in natural healing. As I've mentioned, the ancient masters believed that change is constant and inevitable, and that the ability to adapt well to change is vital for health and longevity. In fact, they thought that physical flexibility was an even more accurate measure of age than chronology. They believed the ability to bend without breaking protected people from many of the assaults that life inflicts.

The great Eastern thinkers said that the universe and all things in it, including our bodies, are forever moving from the yin condition to that of yang, and then back again, in a ceaseless cycle of change. As the philosopher Lao Tzu said, "The ceaseless intermingling of heaven [yang] and earth [yin] gives form to all things." This cycle of change is thought to be as inexorable as the changing seasons, and the cycle of night and day. The constant change is not chaotic, but is orderly and predictable, and infuses all things with energy, just as the changing seasons invigorate and nurture the earth. In the body, this constant change is experienced as the mix of opposing forces that swirls the chakras, and brings the energy of the cosmos into our physical and ethereal selves.

According to Eastern healers, health breaks down when we resist change, and is improved by actions that are in accord with change. For example, ingesting the herb ginseng is considered important in Eastern medicine, because ginseng is a biochemical adaptogen, which helps the body adapt to change. Ginseng does this by improving the health of the adrenal glands. Healthy adrenal glands are important for handling the stress of change, because the adrenals are activated every time we face a challenge and must change our actions accordingly. Without strong adrenals, a person is far more apt to handle change poorly, and to become stressed by it.

But one of the best exercises for developing flexibility in all aspects of life is to develop physical flexibility. Flexibility, particularly of the spine, is important for proper nerve function. If the spinal cord is impinged upon by a stiff and inflexible spinal column, it is less able to neurologically nurture the body. As Yogi Bhajan has stated, "You may die, but you'll never grow old if you have a flexible spine."

An interesting example of this principle was exhibited by my coauthor Cameron Stauth's father, Vernon Stauth. Mr. Stauth was a remarkably energetic man who had an amazing degree of physical flexibility. Every year on his birthday, even after he was seventy, he would perform an astonishing feat of flexibility. Holding a yardstick horizontally behind his back, he would jump through the yardstick—so that it was in front of him—without dropping it. If you try this yourself, be careful, because it's extremely difficult, even for veteran yoga practitioners.

Mr. Stauth had some poor health habits, such as smoking and eating carelessly, but still had the physical power, after his retirement, to build his own home almost single-handedly, and to do all the work on a small farm. However, in his late seventies, he fell off a roof and shattered his heel. During his long convalescence he lost a great deal of his flexibility and fitness, and he soon died. Even his approaching death, though, did not daunt him—possibly because he'd had two separate near-death experiences, and possibly because he'd learned the deepest lessons of flexibility. He saw death as just another change, and accepted it with humor and grace.

Balance

Balance is often derived from flexibility, and is integral to physical, psychological, and spiritual health. When people are flexible, they are able to make the continual series of adjustments that restores balance.

In the Eastern tradition, illness is seen as a result of imbalance. The theory of the Five Elements is based around maintaining balance. If one of the Five Elements is in excess, the opposite element should be stimulated, to restore balance.

From the Western perspective, balance is also considered important to health. Most Western physicians now agree that a lifestyle dominated by imbalanced behaviors presents many risk factors for disease. People who eat too much, work too much, or worry too much are very vulnerable to illness.

Western physicians also generally agree that endocrine imbalance, in particular, often destroys health. The most common condition of endocrine imbalance that ruins health is overproduction of stimulating hormones, such as cortisol and adrenaline, due to stress. When stimulating hormones predominate, they shift the body toward the stimulating fight-or-flight, sympathetic branch of the nervous system, and away from the calming parasympathetic branch. Unfortunately, the calming, rest-and-repair, parasympathetic branch is needed for healing.

Kundalini yoga is especially adept at restoring endocrine balance, by focusing physical and ethereal energies on particular endocrine glands. Long before the advent of modern endocrinology, Eastern healers used kundalini yoga and other forms of yoga to rebalance the endocrine system. The ancient healers used various postures and movements that (1) increased blood circulation to various endocrine glands, and (2) increased the flow of ethereal energy to certain organs and glands. Both of these actions enhanced the secretions of the glands.

One kundalini yoga method of increasing both blood circulation and ethereal energy was to create pressure around a gland. Various postures increase this pressure, and stimulate specific glands. For example, lying on one's back and raising one's legs at different angles affects different endocrine glands. If the legs are raised only slightly, from 0 to 6 inches, it brings pressure to the ovaries and testes, and optimizes their function. If the legs are raised from 12 to 24 inches, it exerts pressure on the liver, spleen, gall bladder, and pancreas, and improves their performance.

Here is the complete table of leg-raise angles that you can use to balance and optimize your own endocrine and organ function.

This pressure, as I noted in the previous chapter, can also be increased with various breathing techniques; as well as with specific energy locks, which I will soon describe.

Other postures and movements that increase flexibility and balance also can improve endocrine function. For example, the very basic movement called Spinal Flex was powerful enough to restore sexual potency to a seventy-year-old patient of mine from Phoenix. This man had gradually become impotent, due primarily to the effects of aging. However, when he began to do the Spinal Flex and a few other yoga exercises, he experienced

ANGLES OF HEALING

The following degrees of leg lift specifically affect the following endocrine glands and organs.

Degree of Lift	Gland or Organ
0–6 inches	Testes, ovaries
0–12 inches	Digestive organs, sex organs and glands, intestines
12 inches–2 feet	Liver, spleen, gall bladder, pancreas
1½ feet–2½ feet	Liver, gall bladder, upper portion of stomach
2–3 feet	Heart, lungs, stomach
4 feet–90 degrees	Thyroid, parathyroid, pineal
90 degrees	Pineal, pituitary, brain

a marked increase in libido and sexual function, as more energy and circulation were directly channeled to his testes and prostate.

Exercises such as the Spinal Flex are not strenuous, nor do they require bending the body into pretzel positions. To do the Spinal Flex you simply sit in the comfortable, legs-crossed position known as Easy Pose (see page 97) and place your hands on your shoulders, with your fingers in front and thumbs behind. You can also sit in a chair. Then you flex your spine forward and backward for two minutes as you inhale and exhale through the nose. Then hold your breath briefly while you direct your mind to bring energy up your spine. As you can see, this one simple exercise uses most of the elements of advanced meditation: posture, movement, hand position, breath, and mental focus. The combination of these synergistic elements, as a kriya, channels both physical and ethereal energy.

Yoga is also especially helpful for restoring the balance to the musculoskeletal system. This, too, is vitally important for health. When the musculoskeletal system is out of balance, it creates a terrible energy drain on the body. For example, imagine how much easier it is to carry two 10-pound buckets of water, one in each hand, than one 20-pound bucket in one hand. The body is created with almost perfect symmetry, but we allow stress, injury, and illness to undermine this symmetry. When this happens, all of our physical tasks—everything from walking to housework—become far more taxing.

In yoga, balance can be restored with two opposing actions: purification (or reduction), and tonification (or addition). Purification actions are performed to reduce excesses. They include fasting, sweating, and emotional catharsis. Purifying yoga musculoskeletal actions include exhalation, forward bends, and some twists. Tonification actions are taken to add strength, and to overcome deficiency. Tonification actions include ingestion of nutrients and herbs, weight resistance exercises, and rest. Tonifying yoga musculoskeletal actions include inhalation, back bends, and shoulder stands.

Conditions of excess are considered to include obesity, irritable bowel syndrome, hypertension, lymphatic congestion, allergies, and anxiety. Conditions of deficiency include chronic fatigue syndrome, low blood pressure, depression, hypoglycemia, AIDS, and hypothyroidism.

Besides helping balance the musculoskeletal system, yoga postures also help balance the meridian system, the nonphysical network of energy conduits that channels *chi* throughout the body. The meridian system is an ethereal counterpart of the nervous system, and it often becomes imbalanced, just as the nervous system often becomes imbalanced. When this occurs, some organs and glands suffer a deficiency of energy, and some have an excess. For example, a deficiency of energy in the liver meridian, combined with an excess of energy in the heart meridian, might result in a condition of hyperactive agitation, with depressed immunity. The corresponding condition in the nervous system would be domination by the sympathetic branch of the nervous system over the parasympathetic branch. This too causes agitation and lowered immunity, by shifting energy away from the rest-and-repair glands and organs and sending it to the fight-or-flight glands and organs.

Even though the meridian system is nonphysical, it strongly impacts the physical aspects of the human body. Similarly, the physical aspects of the human body—including postures and movements—impact the meridian system. For thousands of years, yogic healers have prescribed various postures and movements to change the energy flow of the meridians, and help people heal. I use this approach in my own medical practice.

Recently, for example, I used the same approach to help a distraught young college-age woman recover from anxiety attacks. Many doctors would have simply placed her on an antianxiety, benzodiazepine drug, such as Valium or Xanax, but this would have left the underlying causative element of her disorder intact. Instead I placed the young woman on a program of Medical Meditation that was centered around a kriya for relaxation and metabolism. This kriya produces deep relaxation by stimulating three major meridians—the large intestine meridian, the Triple Heater, and the gall bladder meridian. This stimulation activates the heart chakra and raises the energy of the electromagnetic field to a higher vibration, which induces calmness. From the Western perspective, the postures and movements of this kriya activate the calming, parasympathetic branch of the nervous system, which releases the chemical milieu that produces relaxation. This chemical milieu includes serotonin and the endorphins.

The final element of the body that is balanced by kundalini yoga postures and movements is the peptides. Peptides, as you may recall from chapter 3, are the partial proteins that trigger the actions of the chemicals that Dr. Candace Pert calls molecules of emotion and molecules of information. Peptides are a key part of the biochemical system that Dr. Pert refers to as the second nervous system. They are produced not only in the brain, but throughout the body, and enable the body and brain to, in effect, speak the same language.

Kundalini yoga movements and postures—when combined with breath control—have the ability to affect the quantity and quality of peptide production. This occurs because of increased pressure, enhanced circulation, the stimulation of physical movement, and improved flow of ethereal energy to the specific areas of the body where peptides are produced.

As you can see, the range of effects from the balancing actions of yoga postures and movements is profound. It is precisely because of these effects that yoga has existed for thousands of years as a medical modality. In comparison, it's unlikely that many of the drugs and surgeries that now constitute Western medicine will still be actively used several thousand years from now. Yoga postures and movements are indeed, to use Dr. Herbert Benson's phrase, "medicine that lasts."

Therefore, it is now appropriate to move on to the most practical aspect of this subject: how you can perform the postures and movements that can help change your life. I will begin this by telling you how to perform energy "locks" that effectively channel and control ethereal energy.

The System of Energy Locks

Locks are created by tensing certain muscles, to temporarily arrest the flow of ethereal energy. These locks—or *bhandas*, in the Sanskrit—are a powerful and practical way for you to increase and direct your body's flow of ethereal energy.

As you'll recall from the chapter on breath, prana enters your body primarily when you breathe. This prana not only awakens your kundalini energy but also infuses you with energy and joy. However, just as the air you breathe eventually exits your body, prana also circulates out of your body, back into the cosmos. The prana that you return to the cosmos is called *apana*.

The air you exhale helps cleanse your body, by removing carbon dioxide from your system. Similarly, the exit of apana from your body helps to ethereally purify you, carrying away the stagnant energies that can collect in the system. Thus, prana and apana are the generative and eliminative energies in your ethereal body. They are the positive and negative aspects of the universal energy.

Within your body, prana and apana mix. This mixture of positive energy and negative energy generates an even greater energy, just as the mixture of all opposing forces amplifies energy. The new force that is created by the swirling of prana and apana is tremendously beneficial because it is a neutral energy that induces calmness and helps the mind to be neutral, that is, nonjudgmental, serene, and peaceful. Achieving a neutral mind is one of the greatest benefits of advanced meditation, because the neutral mind is a potent healing force, a key part of the sacred space in which all healing occurs. Achieving this neutral energy within the body also enables prana to awaken your kundalini, which then flows freely from chakra to chakra. It allows energy to move fluidly from the lower chakras to the higher ones, and thus creates a sense of personal power and elevated consciousness.

Postures, movements, and breath control help to mix the prana and apana and direct their flow. So, too, do the kundalini yoga energy locks, or bhandas. The bhandas literally lock prana and apana into specific areas, so that these two opposing forces have the opportunity to meet and merge. The use of bhandas is central to the practice of kundalini yoga, and also certain other forms of yoga. There are three primary bhandas: the root lock (or *mul bhanda*), the diaphragm lock (or *uddiyana bhanda),* and the neck lock (or *jalandhana bhanda).* When all three are applied simultaneously, it creates the great lock (or *mahabhanda).*

THE ROOT LOCK

The root lock is slightly more complicated than the other two locks, but has a powerful effect. It stimulates and circulates the energies of the lower chakras and helps transform sexual energy into creativity and physical regeneration. It can also be used to enhance sexual energy.

The root lock does this by uniting and swirling the energies of prana and apana at the navel center. It directs apana upward from the lower chakras, and directs prana downward from the higher chakras. When these two opposing forces meet, it creates inner heat, or *tapa*, which flows up the *sushmana*, the central nadi through which kundalini energy rises. This tapa also stimulates the movement of kundalini energy up the sushmana. In effect, tapa puts the ethereal form of an electrical charge on the rising kundalini.

To perform the root lock, first contract the anal sphincter, and contract the muscles around the sex organs, as if you were trying to stop the flow of urine. Then contract the muscles around the navel point, and pull them backward, toward the spine. As you do this, the breath may be held in, or out.

THE DIAPHRAGM LOCK

The Sanskrit word for the diaphragm lock, *uddiyana,* means to fly up, and refers to the diaphragm lock's ability to raise energy up from the lower abdomen.

The diaphragm lock raises this lower-chakra energy by helping energy to cross a natural barrier that exists in the lower abdomen—the barrier formed by the muscles of the upper diaphragm, which can sometimes inhibit blood circulation, and also inhibit the flow of ethereal energy. In addition, the barrier reduces the mingling of prana and apana, and beyond the physical, it is considered to be a psychological barrier; the psychic functions below the barrier tend to be unconscious and reactive, while the psychic functions above it are more conscious and flexible.

The diaphragm lock, though, helps ethereal energy and blood circulation to breach this barrier. When this happens, it promotes vertical integration of the opposing qualities above and below the area, by forcing a more complete mixture of prana and apana. This not only helps to balance the psyche but also allows enhanced awakening of the kundalini energy that exists below the barrier. This kundalini energy then flows more forcefully upward, through the central channel of the sushmana.

The diaphragm lock also helps increase the fire energy that emanates from the solar plexus. As this fire energy is increased, it helps open the heart chakra, and magnifies the psychological qualities of compassion and patience.

To apply the diaphragm lock, sit comfortably, inhale deeply, then exhale. Pull your abdomen back toward your spine, and up, as you lift your chest. Gently press your lower back forward. Hold the position for 10 seconds to 1 minute. As you do the lock, try to maintain a feeling of calmness and balance.

THE NECK LOCK

The neck lock is the most fundamental of all bhandas. It is used in many meditations that employ mantras and breath control. Therefore, it is used in many Medical Meditations.

The function of the neck lock is to seal and contain the energy generated in the upper areas of the brain stem. The neck lock exerts a number of physiological effects. It stabilizes blood pressure in the head, which can be disrupted by exercise and breath control. It also heightens blood circulation to the thyroid and parathyroid. Furthermore, it stimulates the pituitary, hypothalamus, and pineal, and enhances the flow of the neuropeptides that enable these endocrine structures to communicate with one another.

The ancient masters described this enhanced endocrinological function as a heightening of the nectars of the brain. They were especially intent upon increasing the secretions of what we now call the pineal gland, and referred to these as the nectar of the moon—an appropriate nomenclature, since the primary hormone secreted by the pineal is melatonin, the hormone that helps us sleep. The ancient masters thought that the nectars of the moon had a cooling effect upon the heated energy that often emanates from the lower chakras.

To apply the lock, sit comfortably with your spine straight. Lift your chest and breastbone upward, and gently pull in your chin, toward the back of your neck. Keep your head level and centered, and keep the muscles of your throat, face, and neck loose.

The locking action of this bhanda is derived primarily from the inward position of the chin.

THE GREAT LOCK

This lock, a combination of the other three, is a general tonifier that has been used for centuries as a curative exercise. It has been used to lower blood pressure, reduce menstrual cramps, improve circulation, improve intestinal function, stimulate nerve function, and improve cognitive energy. Furthermore, it is believed that the great lock helps the body to more fully achieve the sacred space. Often, the great lock is applied at the end of a set of yoga kriyas.

To perform it, inhale and pull the root lock, then exhale and apply all three locks simultaneously, and hold them for 10 seconds to 1 minute. Always end by inhaling, exhaling, and relaxing the breath.

You will notice that a great many of the Medical Meditations use at least one of these locks. Once you've mastered them, you'll find that they magnify the healing energy of your body, and help you to focus this energy where it's needed most.

Yoga Mudras

For thousands of years, yogis have used specific hand and finger positions as an important part of their yoga postures and movements. They believed that hand and finger positions, and movement of the fingers, had a potent effect upon the brain. This belief has been confirmed by a number of medical experiments. Let me tell you about one.

In this experiment, conducted recently by the National Institute of Mental Health, participants performed a finger exercise, while researchers monitored their brains with MRI scans. Then, for several weeks, the participants practiced the exercise, which consisted of touching each of their fingers, one after another, to their thumbs. Finally, researchers monitored participants' brains again while they did the exercise. At the same session, though, the participants also did a finger exercise that they had not practiced.

Researchers noted something that was very interesting and highly promising. Participants used about the same amount of brain activity during the very first brain scan—before they started practicing—as when they performed the new exercise. However, they used significantly more of their brains when they did the exercise that they'd practiced.

This indicated that the repetition of this simple physical task had actually enlarged the capacity of their brains, increasing connections between neurons and forging new neuronal pathways. The researchers concluded that the finger exercise had contributed significantly to brain plasticity, the ability of the brain to renew itself. Most of the renewal had occurred, they found, in the motor cortex of the brain, which controls physical movement. In my own practice, though, I have noted even more far-reaching effects from the regular practice of yoga hand and finger positions—or *mudras,* in the Sanskrit. One thing I've noticed is that mudras improve overall ability to control movement. This is reasonable to expect, since any functional enlargement of the motor-sensory cortex can be expected to increase general physical coordination. More interestingly, though, I've also noted a significant improvement in alertness among patients who regularly practice mudras as part of their Medical Meditations. This seems to indicate that more than just the motor cortex may be stimulated by mudras.

One of my patients, Ronald, used mudras to help combat two serious conditions. One was early-stage Alzheimer's disease, which had begun to muddle his cognitive ability. The other was a marked lack of coordination, due to encephalopathy that had been caused by a deficiency of vitamin B-1. Ronald had been a heavy drinker. This had triggered the B-1 deficiency, which is relatively common among heavy drinkers. He was also prone to depression, agitation, and insomnia.

Before he began Medical Meditation, Ronald was unable to stand up after sitting in a chair, without wobbling. He also couldn't walk well unless his wife held his elbow to steady him. When he first tried to do basic mudras, his finger movements were clumsy and uncertain.

With his wife's help, he worked hard at his mudras, though, and they appeared to have a dramatic effect upon his overall motor abilities. His walking became much steadier, and he didn't have trouble getting out of a chair. Even more gratifying, though, were improvements in his mood and alertness. He felt better emotionally, communicated more fluently, and slept better. As I worked with him, I became convinced that the mudras he practiced were a valuable element of his healing regimen. I believe that they helped to restore millions of neuronal connections.

The power of finger movements to improve the brain may stem from the anatomical fact that control of the hands and fingers requires the use of large areas of the brain. Moving the fingers deftly is neurologically difficult, but vitally important to survival. Therefore, through the force of evolution, the brain has developed an abundance of neurological connections to control finger and hand movement. The following medical illustration, called a homunculus, is a graphic representation of the large area of the brain that is associated with hand movement. As you'll notice, another area of the body that is highly represented in the brain is the tongue. From a neurological perspective, skillful movement of the tongue is quite difficult, and requires billions of neuronal connections. This is the primary reason that the power of speech is one of the last skills babies master.

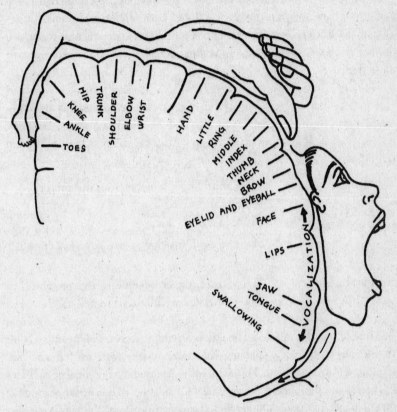

Illustration showing how the fingers, lips, and tongue are highly represented in the brain. (Modeled after Penfield and Rasmussen, *Cerebral Cortex of Man*, The Macmillan Co.)

As you can see in this illustration, some parts of the hand—most notably the thumb—require even more brain space than others. Because of this, your thumb is literally smarter than the rest of your fingers. To prove this to yourself, touch your thumb to your palm, without moving your other fingers.

It's relatively easy. Then touch your index finger to your palm, without moving your other fingers. It's harder, because your index finger is not governed by as many neurological connections as your thumb. Try your other fingers, and you'll find it gets increasingly hard to move only one finger at a time as you work your way toward your little finger. In fact, it's almost impossible to move your little finger to your palm without moving the finger next to it. Your little finger is your least educated finger. Moving it by itself is as hard as wiggling your ears. Yoga masters can do it, but most other people can't.

In the Eastern healing tradition, each of the fingers is also thought to have a symbolic, or archetypal, identity. Here are the archetypal representations.

THUMB	The symbol of divine energy, which has risen above the ego and the material world
INDEX FINGER	The so-called Jupiter finger, which carries the energy of the ego, and the subconscious
MIDDLE FINGER	The Saturn finger, which carries the energy of stability and strength
RING FINGER	The Sun finger, which resonates with the energy of the solar plexus chakra, and governs personal power
LITTLE FINGER	The Mercury finger, which is related to your intellectual and worldly activities

In addition, certain hand positions also have archetypal meanings. One of the most obvious is placing the palms open, with your hands outstretched in front of you. This symbolizes openness, friendliness, and lack of threat, and has been used by almost all cultures in the world as a sign of greeting and affection. Another archetypal sign is placing the hands together in front of you, palms touching, fingertips upraised, in prayer position. In a multitude of cultures, this signifies respect and humility.

These archetypal meanings are also thought to help create the feelings that they symbolize. Simply doing these simple, archetypal hand positions helps to change a person's outlook. Just opening your palms and reaching out helps you to feel more open and receptive.

Following are some of the most common mudras. You will use them in many of your Medical Meditations.

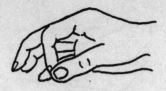

GYAN MUDRA

The tip of the index finger touches the tip of the thumb. This is the mudra of wisdom, because it joins the divine finger with the finger of self. This signifies an awareness of the illusion of the ego, without an abandonment of the self.

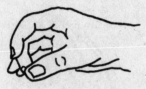

SHUNI MUDRA

The tip of the middle finger touches the tip of the thumb. This gesture confers patience.

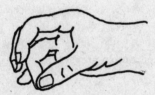

SURYA MUDRA

The tip of the ring finger (symbolized as Uranus or the Sun) touches the tip of the thumb, giving energy, health, intuition.

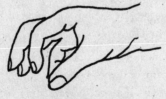

BUDDHI MUDRA

The tip of the little finger (Mercury) touches the tip of the thumb. This helps bring clear and intuitive communication.

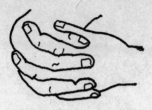

VENUS LOCK MUDRA

Interlace the fingers with the right little finger on the bottom. The left thumb is on top. During meditation, this mudra helps people to maintain focus and concentration. The instructions for proper placement of this mudra will be given when utilized for a specific Medical Meditation.

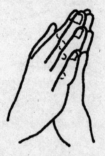

PRAYER MUDRA

The palms are flat together, which helps the yin and yang to be neutralized. This is used for centering, and in preparation for doing a kriya.

Let's start with the most basic postures, or poses. You will use them in many of your Medical Meditations. Always remember to tune in by chanting "Ong Namo Guru Dev Namo" before kundalini yoga or meditation. Now let's put all this information on flexibility, balance, kriyas, energy locks, and mudras together, as I show you some of the most valuable and revered yoga postures and movements.

Fundamental Postures and Movements

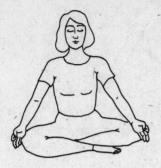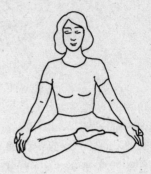

EASY POSE

There are three variations of Easy Pose, the most commonly used posture in Medical Meditation.

1. Sit cross-legged, with the feet tucked in under the opposite knees. Pull the spine up straight and press the lower spine slightly forward.
2. Sit with the legs out straight. Pull one foot in next to the groin. Place the other foot over the ankle of the first foot, so that it rests near the thigh. Straighten the spine. This is the Half Lotus variation. It is more difficult than the first variation.
3. This is like the first variation, but the top foot is placed on the calf of the other leg, rather than right at the groin. In this pose, make sure to press the lower spine forward, as it will have a tendency to slip backward.

All these variations of Easy Pose are easier than Lotus Pose, and require less flexibility. The drawback is that one must be more conscious of keeping the lower spine slightly forward, so the upper spine can stay straight. If you cannot sit cross-legged on the floor, you may sit straight in a chair.

LOTUS POSE

Sit with the legs extended forward. Spread the legs. Bend the left leg so the left heel comes to the groin. Lift the left foot onto the upper right thigh.

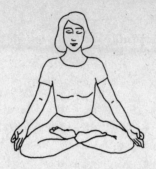

Bend the right leg so that the right foot rests on top of the left thigh, as close to the abdomen as possible. Straighten the spine. Lift the chest and press the lower spine slightly forward. In this position you will feel locked in place. Once you are in it, you can meditate very deeply, and the position will maintain itself.

Although very few of the exercises or Medical Meditations in this book require this difficult posture, it is recognized as one of the best postures for deep meditation.

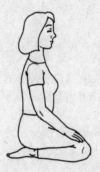

ROCK POSE

This posture is well known for its beneficial effects on the digestive system. It gained its nickname from the idea that one who masters the posture can sit in it and digest rocks. It also makes you as solid and balanced as a rock. It is used in many kundalini yoga kriyas, but is rarely used by itself.

To get in the position, start by kneeling on both knees, with the tops of the feet on the ground. Sit back on the heels. The heels will press two nerves that run into the lower center of each buttock. Keep the spine straight.

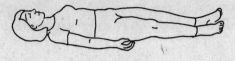

CORPSE POSE

Lie flat on your back, with your arms along your sides and your palms facing up. The archetypal meaning of Corpse Pose is that of dying to old ways of thinking and moving. Also, as you lie on the floor, it enables you to perceive the boundaries of your body as they merge with the floor and you enter into the desired state of neutrality. Yoga masters say that the Corpse Pose feels like nothing. It is the perfect posture for total relaxation after yoga or meditation, or before sleep.

Medical Meditation to Generate Healing Energy
(See also first chakra, page 176)

This Medical Meditation, also called Sat Kriya, is one of the most powerful kriyas in the science of kundalini yoga. With regular practice, it increases lung capacity, perfects the functioning of the organs, stimulates circulation, generates great energy, and raises kundalini energy up the spine.

I practice it daily for at least 3 minutes, and frequently prescribe it to patients. At 11 minutes, it is a complete kriya. During advanced white tantric yoga, it can be done for 31 minutes to 3 hours. In fact, I know practitioners who have done Sat Kriya for 2½ hours a day for 40 days. This takes people to a whole new level of energy.

Sitting on the heels, with a straight spine, stretch the arms straight up overhead, hugging the ears. Interlace the fingers, with the index fingers pressed together and pointing straight up. The eyes are closed and focused at the third-eye point.

Chant "Sat" (rhymes with "but") as you apply the root lock. Release the lock as you chant "Nam" (rhymes with "mom"). Your breath will come automatically. Do this in a consistent rhythm of approximately eight times per 10 seconds.

Continue for at least 3 minutes. Then inhale, hold the breath, and exhale deeply several times. On the last exhalation, hold the air out and apply the great lock. Focus on moving energy up your spine to your third-eye point. Inhale, and squeeze the lower-back muscles tightly, all the way from the buttocks to the back, mentally urging the energy to flow up to the top of the skull.

Lie on your back and rest, for approximately as long as you performed the exercise.

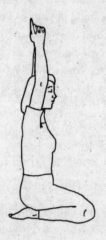

CHAPTER SIX

Mantra

The Tides and Rhythms

of the Universe

In the City of Immortality, everything was vibrating. The heat cast a shimmering pulse over the landscape, and nothing was still, not even my soul. I was on edge, expectant. What would happen next on this journey? A miracle? A disaster?

I was crushed among a throng of people, pressed so closely to them that I could actually feel their heartbeats. In India—the site of the City of Immortality, or Amritsar—there is no sense of personal space. To get a better view of Amritsar's Golden Temple, people will literally climb right on top of you. But they'll also find a way to squeeze you in, if you're left out.

Oddly, the sensation of the heartbeats around me seemed somehow to merge, and to beat in unison, until finally there was only one pulse. I could feel my own heart begin to synchronize with this beat. It was powerful, but unsettling. I was a stranger in a strange land. Held so tightly in this grip of humanity, I was losing my sense of what was flesh and what was fantasy.

My disorientation had begun long before I arrived at this sacred place. Separated from home by thousands of miles, many time zones, and incalculable cultural differences, I'd boarded a plane earlier in the morning that had taken me from New Delhi to Amritsar. On the plane was a group of tourists, prototypical Ugly Americans wearing plaid shorts and golf shirts, with cameras around their necks, intent upon getting the 25-cent tour of the holy hot spots: first the Golden Temple in the City of Immortality, and then a quick bus run up the road to Dharmsala, the Place of Truth, where the Dalai Lama lived. Then lunch, then shopping. Then dinner, then back to the New Delhi Hyatt, for CNN and the stock quotes. One man, in particular, seemed to represent all the materialistic, rationalistic Westernism I'd tried to leave behind on this spiritual pilgrimage. He was wearing a light blue polo shirt and tan slacks, and was talking a mile a minute about all the places he'd been, all the places he was going, and all the stuff he'd bought. He gave the impression that he'd seen it all—and experienced nothing.

My initial reaction to him was: Thank God I'm not like this guy. But the more I thought about it, the more I wondered if I were really that different from him. After all, by judging and categorizing him, wasn't I playing the same games of status and superficiality that I presumed he was?

After we landed, I got another bracing dose of self-realization. My wife, Kirti, and I took a brief bus tour to a small temple in Bakala, where the great guru Teg Bahadur had meditated hundreds of years before. The guru had spent twenty-seven years in a dark basement in his mother's home, meditating upon the nature of God. According to the spiritual literature, he had become enlightened, and had then emerged from the basement and helped bring others to enlightenment. To commemorate him, a small temple had been built over his basement.

The tour guide, a fierce, wiry, warrior-class man carrying a sword and a dagger, began to tell the story of Guru Teg Bahadur. I raised my hand. In typical American fashion, I wanted to know the who-what-where-when-how of this legend. I wanted the practical details—the how-to—that would make the guru's feat of more personal value, something I could take home and use.

"What was the mantra that Guru Teg Bahadur chanted?" I asked the tour guide.

His eyes began to expand, almost explode. "The what?"

"The mantra. What did he say?"

"You do not believe this!" he shouted.

"No, no, don't take me wrong. I'm just curious. I just want to *know* more. To understand."

"Get out!" He was furious. "Get out! Get out!"

In my mind, I saw him reaching for his sword. I saw him lopping off my head in a mighty swing. I saw the headlines in the Indian press: "Infidel Meets Justice." And in the American press: "Minor Incident at Temple; Ambassador Apologizes."

I scooted away, red-faced. Why couldn't I just absorb the powerful vibrations of this sacred place, and put a lid on my researching?

I entered the small temple, and was drawn immediately to the doorway of the basement, where Guru Teg Bahadur had meditated. Suddenly, for no explicable reason, my emotional self-involvement vanished, as if nothing could have been more trivial, and a sense of peace swept over me. At that moment, nine words came to my mind in a language that I do not speak. In Gurumukhi, an ancient spiritual language derived from Sanskrit, I said, "Dhan Dhan Guru Teg Bahadur Sahib Ji Wahe Guru" ("Honored and adorned is Guru Teg Bahadur; ecstasy is in the light of God").

I have no idea how I spoke a language I don't know. It had never happened before, and I don't expect it to happen again.

I closed my eyes, and more words came into my mind: "Har Har Wahe Guru" ("God's name takes you from darkness to light").

"Har Har Wahe Guru. Har Har Wahe Guru." A current of electricity shot up my spine.

I did not feel as if I were speaking the words, but as if the words were speaking me. My heart and soul went to a quiet place that was without time or space.

After what seemed like just a moment, I felt the essence of Kirti around me, though I heard nothing and saw nothing. I slowly opened my eyes. She was there.

"The bus is leaving," she said.

"What about the tour here?"

"Everyone's seen it. We've been here a long time."

I repeated the mantra one more time, bowed in reverence to this holy man, and left.

The mantra I had been saying was, it turned out, the very mantra that Guru Teg Bahadur had used hundreds of years before.

I do not know, to this day, exactly how I knew that mantra, nor how I knew those words in Gurmuki, except to think that it was a gift from the guru. I do clearly recall, though, that as I left Bakala, I had a profound feeling of peace, and a heightened sensation of intuition.

I carried this sense of peace and awareness with me to the Golden Temple. But as the crowd began to close in around me, and as the heat and sun began to vibrate my surroundings like a mirage, my analytic mind again emerged and I became restless. What I mostly wanted to know was, Where were the healings? The small lake in front of the Golden Temple was renowned as a body of healing water, and I hoped to observe some people bathe in the water, or drink it, and be healed of their illness. I had heard many stories of healing miracles occurring here, even to people who had no faith in the water. The Golden Temple, the geographic center of the Sikh religion, is as famous for healing in the East as Lourdes is in the West. It holds a special spiritual energy, as do places such as the Wailing Wall, Mecca, Jerusalem, and the Vatican. The City of Immortality and the City of Truth, so close together, are a vortex of ethereal power. As a medical doctor, I longed to see this power expressed in a positive medical outcome. After all, seeing, as they say, is believing.

According to legend, this lake was the place where a young woman came, long ago, seeking refuge. The woman, daughter of a king, met a leper, saw the man behind the disfigurement, and fell in love with him. The king had warned her not to marry him, but she did, and they were ostracized. When they came to the lake, the man accidentally fell into the water. When he emerged, the woman did not recognize him. He did not have leprosy. He protested that he was her husband, but she did not believe him. Then he raised his hand, which had not been immersed, and it was still leprotic. He dipped his hand in the water, and it was healed.

From that time on, people began to come to the lake for healing. During the sixteenth century, Guru Ram Das, the Fourth Master of the Sikh religion, had built a temple by the healing water, and it eventually became the Golden Temple, a beautiful edifice of marble and gold. The Golden Temple had doors on all four sides and was open to everyone, in outright defiance of India's caste system.

In this place, people now come to cleanse their karma and find their highest selves. They come to wash away the sins of their souls. Surrounding me were Sikhs, Muslims, Hindus, Buddhists, Christians, spiritualists, and tourists. From a distance, I even saw the American in the blue shirt. Everyone wanted to enter the temple, but few could squeeze in. The crowd pressed against my chest, stifling my breath. The claustrophobia was overpowering. There was no way to get to a drinking fountain, a restroom, or a piece of shade.

Where were the healings? I craned my neck. What could I learn here that might help my patients or myself?

Then the chanting began. A group of three singers, or *ragis*, began to play their instruments and sing at the base of the temple, about thirty yards away. They were singing a mantra: "Wahe Guru, Wahe Guru, Wahe Guru, Wahe Jio." It was very simple, very beautiful, and heartfelt: "The God in my soul takes me from darkness to light."

The three singers were dressed in immaculate matching blue *bana,* traditional Indian outfits with ornate turbans. One played a tabla, a linked treble and bass drum, and the other two were playing harmoniums, accordion-like keyboards.

The crowd took up the mantra, hundreds of voices in harmony, and it created an overwhelming vibration. The vowel sounds were elongated, and this contributed powerfully to the vibratory effects of the words. From every side of me, and from above and below, I could feel the vibrations of sound enter my body. The earth seemed to tremble. As I joined in the mantra, I created an even more pronounced vibration in my own skull. I focused on my third-eye point and felt the vibrations touch my brain.

All sound, of course, is vibration. The ears create sound from this vibration, but even without ears, there is still vibration. Every moment of the day, everywhere we are, the energy vibrations that can create sound travel through us, vibrating every cell in our bodies. Even in the vacuum of space, sound waves vibrate to the outer recesses of the universe, toward infinity.

In the human body, the vibratory waves that can cause sound have their most pronounced effect upon our two most sensitive systems: the neurological and the endocrine systems. The vibrations that we create ourselves, through our own speech, have the most direct, powerful effects. They strongly vibrate the brain, as well as the pituitary and hypothalamus, which are located near the roof of the mouth.

When this occurs, wondrous physiological actions take place. Vibrating the pituitary, the master gland of the endocrine system, notably increases the function of that gland, just as massaging a lymph gland potentiates the function of the lymph gland. Vibrating the pituitary increases its output of secretions, and this in turn optimizes the function of the entire endocrine system.

The vibratory effects of chanting also have several other important physical actions.

1. They improve immune function, via the hypothalamic-pituitary axis.
2. They increase brain hemispheric balance.

3. They send ethereal energy coursing through the nadis.
4. They help quiet the inner dialogue.
5. They help potentiate the proper replication of DNA, thus helping maintain generic integrity.

Furthermore, the meaning of the mantras penetrates the psyche, creating tremendous psychoactive healing power.

Many of these positive effects occur because of the particular sound patterns and vocal movements that specific mantras create. The ancient mantras, some of which are thousands of years old, were chosen specifically because of the sounds within them. On the simplest level, these sounds include a plethora of vowels, which create much greater vibratory actions than percussive consonants. However, certain consonants also have strong, direct actions, because of the way they make the tongue strike the upper palate. This striking force is carried to the pituitary, which is only millimeters away from the upper palate.

Because of these many potent effects, the chanting of mantras, or specific phrases, has been an important part of the spiritual practices of virtually all cultures, throughout the world, throughout history. The Catholic religion employs the chanting of many repetitive prayers, such as the Hail Mary. Chanting is an important part of the Jewish cabalistic tradition. Native Americans centered many of their religious rituals around chanting. Buddhists and Sufis chant mantras, and Muslims use repetitive prayers. Chanting is also central to the religious practices of such far-flung and disparate cultures as the New Guinea Melanesians, the Australian aborigines, and the African Mbutis. This universal acceptance of vibratory sound as a spiritual conduit is, I believe, strongly indicative of its intrinsic power.

As I chanted outside Amritsar's Golden Temple, I began to feel a shift in my state of mind, due to a subtle rearrangement of my endocrinological secretions, and neurochemistry. I definitely felt stimulated, as if I'd just drunk a couple of cups of coffee, but at the same time I didn't feel any agitation or restlessness.

In this heightened condition of consciousness, I began to pray. I prayed for the safety of my children, for the health of my patients, and for the success of my nonprofit organization, the Alzheimer's Prevention Foundation. These prayers felt powerful, as if they could become reality just by my imagining them. Still, though, these prayers didn't seem to fully resonate with the vibration that permeated this holy place. I stopped my prayers of petition, or intercessionary prayers, and focused solely upon the nature of the divine spirit, and how happy I was to be a part of that spirit. As I did this, my meditation deepened, time fell away, and I lost sense of where my own body ended and the bodies around me began. My prayer became very simple: "Let the right thing happen. May all blessings come. Thy will be done." Somehow, this prayer seemed to mesh perfectly with the atmosphere surrounding me.

For precious moments—or maybe an hour or two, I really don't know—I felt as if I were the crowd, and the crowd was me, and that we were all speaking in one voice. The sound vibrations entering my brain and body felt very tactile, as if they had shape and form.

On a purely physical level, my hormones, neurotransmitters, and neuropeptides were dancing in perfect synchronization. The nodal-point hot spots of neuropeptides throughout my body seemed to be vibrating in harmony with my brain and my breath. As you may recall, the systemic neuropeptides communicate with one another and with the brain, not through a lock-and-key system, as long presumed, but through a system of harmonic, interlocking vibrations.

My cognitive power, mood, and energy continued to elevate, borne on a rising tide of endocrine and neurotransmitter release. I felt simultaneously relaxed and invigorated, as if I could either run a marathon or go to sleep. More than anything else, I felt as I had felt as a child, when energy was endless and joy was my usual state of mind.

I lifted my head in happiness and saw hawks and swallows swooping in flight. I could not see the air that supported them, but I could clearly see the support the air offered, as the birds beat their wings against it. At that moment, the air seemed as tangible as the sound currents that were buzzing through my body.

I heard a splashing, sloshing noise, and a cry of ecstasy. Perhaps someone had plunged into the healing waters and been relieved of suffering. But I was too transfixed by the birds to look.

Watching the birds, I suddenly experienced a certainty that there was an invisible force supporting me—supporting all of us—just as surely as the air was supporting the birds. Throughout my body—not just in my brain— a realization took shape: There is one, true, immortal essence of reality who is the doer of all things.

This did not feel like a thought. It felt like an experience. It did not feel like something I had learned. It felt like something I had become.

"Wahe Guru, Wahe Guru, Wahe Guru, Wahe Jio. Wahe Guru, Wahe Guru, Wahe Guru, Wahe Jio." My words seemed to take form, and fly, like birds, to the sky: "The God in my soul takes me from darkness to light."

At some point, I entered the temple. I remember the exquisite feeling that descended upon me. Since that day, this feeling has been with me. Sometimes, during moments of stress or fatigue, it blurs and softens. But it's part of me now, as intrinsic to my being as the color of my eyes.

On my way out of the temple, I saw an elderly man pressing his forehead against the temple, chanting fervently. The temple seemed still to vibrate. But the heat was gone. If there was a vibration, its source was far more ethereal than that of mere heat.

As I reveled in this magical convergence of time and place, watching the old man meditate, I again saw the American from the airplane. He was emerging from the temple. But he seemed quite different. Or maybe I was just seeing him with different eyes. He was no longer fast and frantic, but was moving with grace and the utmost deliberation. He had placed a kerchief over his head, in reverence. His eyes were fixed, and there seemed to be a gloss of tears in them. That was not unusual; many people weep here, even the tourists. Somehow, though, this man was no longer just a tourist. In a very real way, he had unexpectedly arrived at his destination.

As he slowly walked past me, he looked into my eyes, and smiled with what seemed to be great kindness. I bowed before him. He bowed back. He was, after all, God. And so were we all, in that time and place. And so are we all, now.

When I returned home, I met with my teacher, Yogi Bhajan. When he first saw me, he looked at me closely. He said, "Your heart has opened." It was true. I had gone to the Golden Temple hoping to see a healing. I had received more than my hopes had held. It was I who had been healed.

The Age of Aquarius

On the first hour of November 11, 1991, the world changed forever. At that moment, the Age of Pisces ended, and the Age of Aquarius began. The transition, governed by a twenty-one-year cusp, will be fully completed in 2012. The ramifications of this shift, however, are already becoming evident.

The single most significant characteristic of the Age of Aquarius is that it revolves around information. The preceding 2,000-year cycle of time, the Age of Pisces, was dominated by machines and hierarchies. The Piscean era, during which mankind created technology, was the age of ego, isolation, and conflict. The Aquarian Age, in contrast, is an era of knowledge, communication, sharing, and experience.

There are, of course, many obvious physical manifestations of our current Age of Information—everything from the egalitarian Internet to the instant transmission of knowledge through fiber-optic communications.

While it is now widely accepted that this is indeed the Age of Information, most people assume that this description of our era arose only after the advent of certain technological innovations, such as the personal computer. In the spiritual literature, though, the modern ascendancy of information was foreseen many hundreds of years ago.

Because times are changing, we must change—just as we must change every time summer turns to winter, and winter to spring. If we fail to change, we will face destruction, in much the same way we would be destroyed if we failed to adjust to the cold of winter. As you'll recall from the chapter on posture and movement, flexibility, literally and in the abstract, is vital to survival.

Our primary challenge as we enter the Age of Aquarius is to adjust to this monumental change in a positive way. The information that is rapidly becoming available to us can be our best friend, or our worst enemy, depending upon how we use it. Thus it is important that we carefully nurture our brains and our psyches, so that we will make the right choices as we swim in this vast sea of information. The information that we are becoming exposed to could solve all of mankind's problems, or destroy humanity forever.

Because of this astonishing new opportunity, it is critically important to furnish the brain and the psyche with a technology that will propel us toward positive choices. One of the most beneficial technologies available to us is that of the science of sound. The ancient masters called this science the Shabd Guru, from *shabd* (pronounced "SHAW-bud"), "sound," and *guru,* "teacher." Thus, the Shabd Guru consists of sounds that teach.

In one of his most profound works, the *Level One Teacher's Manual,* psychologist and yoga master Gurucharan Singh Khalsa, Ph.D., describes the complete etiology of Shabd Guru. *Shabd,* he notes, comes from *sha,* "ego," and *bd,* "to shut off." *Gu* means darkness, and *ru* means light. Thus, the transformational *shabd,* or sound, is composed of sounds that shut off the ego, and take us from darkness to light.

The ego, in this usage, refers not simply to the most common, narrow meaning of the word, "vanity," but to the personal entity that is formed when the mind attaches itself to, and identifies with, various objects, feelings, and thoughts. This isolated, self-involved ego is not inherently bad. In fact, it's absolutely human. But it's limited—terribly limited.

When people believe that the ego aspect of their being represents their entire being, they set themselves up for suffering. If you believe that your ego is all that you are, then you are vulnerable, first and foremost, to fear of death. You are also vulnerable to all other forms of material suffering, such as disease, financial distress, and humiliation. If you think you're nothing but your materialistically attached ego, then you're missing out on the greatest opportunity in your life—the chance to experience your own godliness. Feeling your own spark of divine energy is the most exciting, pleasurable, and empowering feeling imaginable.

The Shabd Guru helps you rise above your ego and come to full consciousness of your own divinity. Therefore it is an indispensable technology for the Aquarian Age. It consists of using words to reach the ultimate word, or vibration—the existence of God.

Imagine, for a moment, that the biblical phrase, "In the beginning was the Word," were to read, "In the beginning was the Vibration." As I've mentioned, all words and sounds are vibration, and all vibration can create sound. Therefore, from the perspective of physics, it can be accurate to use "word" and "vibration" interchangeably. According to this logic, it is meaningful to perceive the creation of the universe in the beginning, as the creation of vibration. After all, every atom in the universe is vibrating, and this vibration is the ultimate animating energy. There could be no life without it. Thus, the Creator might be conceived of as the force that has set this vibration into motion. Of course, the organization of this vibration into the patterns and rhythms of the universe necessarily implies intelligence and intention. The universe does not vibrate randomly, or discordantly; on earth and in the heavens, all vibrations are rhythmic, patterned, and predictable. This is seen in everything from the ocean tides to the vibrations of subatomic particles.

Because the force of vibration is so intricately bound to the core of our being, not just any words will put us in touch with the universal vibrations, or the tides and rhythms of eternity. If you use the wrong sounds and the wrong words, nothing will happen. As Dr. Gurucharan has noted, if you are calling out for God, but get mixed up and instead call out "dog," your dog will come, God won't.

The proper, effective words and sounds, distilled over many centuries, are largely derived from the ancient practice of *naad* yoga, the yoga of sound. Many thousands of years ago the ancient yoga masters, whom many believed to be divinely inspired, selected special sounds that resonate and harmonize with the innate vibrations of the universe. As I stated earlier, these special sounds have specific physiological effects. They increase the brain's ability to operate at a higher level of intuition, perception, and cognition. They heighten the function of the neurological components that make spiritual perception possible.

In the Age of Aquarius, we must begin to use words differently to achieve the things we want from life. In the Age of Pisces, characterized by ego and attachment, words could successfully manipulate the material world to fulfill the needs of the individual. But this way of using words will simply not work in the Aquarian era. In our new age, we must speak from the heart, not the ego. We must stop calculating what we can get with our words. We must, in effect, learn a new language.

The language we must learn is the language of the Shabd Guru. As Dr. Gurucharan Singh has written, "In the beginning, you recite the Shabd Guru in order to clear the mind, and attain awareness. When you reach a state of mastery, you still recite the Shabd because you have become the Shabd, and the Shabd has become you." In essence, you reach the point where you allow the Doer of all things to arrange your affairs. This is the highest form of the colloquial phrase, "Go with the flow." It is healing in action.

If you have not studied the science of sound, you might feel as if this emphasis on its power is overstated. Therefore, let's take a little deeper look into the effect of sound, and see what scientists and physicians say about it.

The Science of Sound

The Greek mathematician Pythagoras was the first prominent early scientist to examine the nature of sound and vibration. Pythagoras believed, with notable prescience, that all forms of matter in the universe emit vibration, from the most distant stars to the smallest particles on earth: "All these sounds and vibrations form a universal harmony, in which each element, while having its own function and character, contributes to the whole." In his most poetic description of the relationship between sound and matter he wrote, "A stone is frozen music."

Pythagoras also believed that sound, and particularly music, could be a powerful healing mechanism. Pythagoras called certain chants, rhythms, and melodies "musical medicine." He applied specific sounds against particular disease conditions, and was so successful that subsequent practitioners followed his protocols for hundreds of years.

Almost 2,500 years after Pythagoras, quantum physicists have proven that the ancient mathematician was correct—all entities in the universe do emit vibrations, however subtle they may be. Physicist Fritjof Capra, in *The Tao of Physics,* wrote, "Rhythmic patterns appear throughout the universe, from the very small to the very large. Atoms are patterns of probability waves, molecules are vibrating structures, and living organisms manifest multiple, interdependent patterns of fluctuations."

Another prominent quantum physicist, Michio Kaku, compared solid matter to the different tones produced by the strings of a violin. He notes, "The answer to the ancient question, 'What is matter?' is simply that matter consists of particles that are different nodes of vibration of the string, such as the note G or F. The 'music' created by the string is matter itself."

Chanting expert Dr. Robert Gass has also contributed significantly to this perspective. "Sound is a remarkable bridge between the two worlds," he writes, "a bridge between spirit and matter. Through the vibrating energy that is sound, the invisible world can reach out and touch this physical plane."

One of the most provocative experiments done on the universality and ubiquity of sound was performed by Dr. Jeffrey Thompson, director of the Center for Neuroacoustic Research in California. Dr. Thompson made a series of tape recordings of various environmental and organic sounds, such as wind, waves, human voices, and animal sounds. He then broke down these sounds electronically, until only the basic primal rhythms and tones remained. He began to play these recordings to patients during a type of healing he calls sonic induction therapy, which appears to promote systemic balance and cellular regeneration.

At one point, a NASA official heard one of the recordings, and was fascinated by it. The NASA official had worked on the exploration projects of the *Voyager I* and *II* spacecrafts, which had traversed the solar system and made audio recordings in deep space. These tapes recorded the vibratory patterns emitted by various planets and moons. Astonishingly, many of the deep space recordings sounded almost exactly like Dr. Thompson's recordings. When Dr. Thompson played the NASA tapes back-to-back with his own recordings, he was struck by the incredible similarities of tone and rhythm. This evidence did indeed appear to indicate that there are universal, primordial sounds that pervade the entire universe.

One possible reason for the similarities of sound patterns throughout the universe may be due to the principle called entrainment, the ability of one vibration to affect another. For example, if one tuning fork is set to a particular vibration, another tuning fork near it will pick up the vibration itself. Similarly, if two pendulums near each other are set into motion, they will soon begin to swing in the same rhythm. This principle even extends to living things. For example, if two muscle cells from the heart are extracted, each will initially pulse to its own rhythm. However, if they are placed closely together, they will each begin to beat with the exact same rhythm.

Another scientific principle that encourages the merging of sounds is resonance. Each object has its own natural frequency of vibration, and when one vibration strikes an object with a similar vibration, the two objects begin to resonate, or vibrate together harmoniously. Also, each will vibrate more forcefully. In music, resonance creates many new, beautiful tones. For example, when the low tones of a violin meet the low tones of a piano, a new, powerful, resonant tone is created that is audible to the human ear.

In general, small objects resonate with high-pitched sounds, while large objects resonate with low-pitched sounds. One of the most striking examples of resonance is the shattering of a crystal glass when a high-pitched sound resonates with the natural frequency of the delicate glass.

Various parts of the human body also resonate with specific sound frequencies. Certain body cavities, such as the sinus cavities, resonate with particular tones and frequencies. High pitches tend to resonate with smaller cavities and structures, and low pitches resonate with larger cavities and structures. Because of this, certain words and sounds have direct effects upon different areas of the body, and can therefore be used therapeutically.

The therapeutic use of sound in modern, Western medicine is still a relatively new endeavor. However, certain ultrasound techniques are well accepted. For example, high-pitched sounds are now sometimes used to disintegrate foreign objects in the body, such as gallstones, and ultrasound scalpels are sometimes used in brain surgery. Sound is also widely used in imaging techniques, such as the ultrasound photos of unborn babies in utero.

Some modern Western physicians have begun to use sound vibration in more innovative ways. The prominent neurologist and author Oliver Sacks, M.D., has found that music therapy can reverse or retard some of the loss of motor skills due to Parkinson's disease. Also, at Yale University, music therapy has been used in certain cases to overcome many of the isolating symptoms of autism.

Researcher Alfred Tomatis has shown that sound can be used therapeutically to treat nervous system disorders. His research indicates that high-pitched sounds energize the nervous system—or charge it, as he says—while low-pitched sounds discharge nervous system energy. This type of sound therapy has been used successfully in the treatment of neurological injury, sleep disorders, and learning disabilities.

Human cells respond in remarkable ways to sound. In one fascinating experiment, cancer cells were exposed for 21 minutes to the sound vibrations of various musical instruments, and to a human voice. As more notes and tones were added, the cancer cells began to destabilize and disintegrate. The most effective sound against the cancer cells was a human voice, singing a musical scale. When applied to healthy cells, though, sound vibration appears to have positive effects. Research has shown that healthy cells exhibit, among other effects, improved oxygen metabolism when exposed to sound.

Because of the powerful effects that sound exerts upon living organisms, researchers have cataloged the positive medical results achieved by chanting and singing, which include:

- Lowered heart rate
- Lowered blood pressure
- Reduction of stress hormones
- Improved output of melatonin
- Increased lymphatic circulation
- Enhanced release of endorphins
- Increased immune system function
- Increased production of interleukin-1

Although some skeptics have argued that sound therapy may have only a psychological effect, Dr. Robert Gass points out that sound has a similarly salutary effect upon animals and even plants. For example, playing certain audiotapes to plants can dramatically increase their uptake of nutrients. In one experiment, an ordinary houseplant exposed to sound began to voraciously soak up nutrients, and grew more than 1,300 feet in length. In the 1973 book by Peter Tompkins and Christopher Bird, *The Secret Life of Plants,* it was inferred that plants could somehow "hear" music, but that makes no sense, because plants don't have ears. It is, of course, the vibration that plants respond to.

As you can see, the power of sound and its efficacy as a new medical modality have been clearly established. Now let's briefly look at why the chanting of certain sounds has such a marked physical effect.

The Physiology of the Shabd Guru

THE HYPOTHALAMIC-PITUITARY AXIS

It was long ago determined by the ancient masters of naad yoga, the yoga of sound, that there are eighty-four reflex points on the upper palate of the mouth, connected to the nearby pituitary and hypothalamus by nonphysical energy channels that are similar to acupuncture meridians. The illustration on page 29 indicates the position of these eighty-four reflex points.

When the tongue forcefully strikes these points, it sends energy through the energy channels, just as inserting an acupuncture needle influences the energy of acupuncture meridians. When this occurs, it stimulates the pituitary and hypothalamus, and this alters the function of the neurological and endocrine systems.

The changes caused by this stimulation can help people in many ways. For more than twenty-five years, the American-based Kundalini Research Institute has documented the effects of vibratory neurological and endocrinological stimulation achieved through the chanting of mantras. Their research indicates that the technology of the Shabd Guru has enabled people to recover from a wide range of conditions, including addiction to drugs and alcohol, depression, anxiety, chronic fatigue, neurosis, and sexual dysfunction.

As you probably remember, the hypothalamus directs the function of the pituitary, and the pituitary in turn governs the function of the entire endocrine system. The endocrine system produces the hormones and neuropeptides that control mood, energy, sexuality, and immunity.

The modern adaptations of the ancient mantras that I will soon present contain the specific words that make the tongue strike these eighty-
four reflex points. In addition, the mantras also produce certain breath patterns, which also influence brain and endocrine function. Working in
harmony, breath, rhythm, and sound produce very specific effects upon
brain chemistry, and upon systemic body chemistry. For example, certain
mantras have the power to stimulate, while others sedate, and some
mantras were specifically designed to heighten immunity, while others were
designed to optimize cognitive function.

As Dr. Gurucharan Singh has written, "If Shabd and breath is the conductor, you are still the composer. You can change the notes, to create
chords of happiness or sadness, to bring the instruments to a rising
crescendo, or to lull them with gentle melodies. The templates of Shabd
Guru are tools for composition. They can write a grand symphony or a
playful jingle. They can create feelings of joy, enthusiasm, or calmness."

When you chant a mantra, you naturally tend to focus upon the meaning of the mantra, such as "God takes me from darkness to light." The meaning of the mantra is powerful, and can trigger a strong physical effect. However, the purely physical action of saying the words is even more powerful
than their meaning. As Gurucharan says, "If you try to maintain a state of
mind by holding one thought, it is very difficult. The thought is slippery, and
is joined by hundreds of competing thoughts. But if you stimulate the hypothalamic conductor to set the state of the body-mind, it is like picking up a
frequency on the radio, or a channel on the TV. In that mode, certain
thoughts are easy to hold, and others are excluded automatically."

One of the most beneficial effects of manipulating the brain and
endocrine system with the Shabd Guru is the improvement that occurs in
the immune response. When the endocrine system and hypothalamus stimulate the healing, rest-and-repair branch of the autonomic nervous system
(the parasympathetic branch), immunity is naturally heightened. In addition, the stimulation of the endocrine system and hypothalamus also
increases other important elements of immunity, such as the production
of natural killer cells that attack viruses. This occurs through the actions of
immunotransmitters, which are guided by the hypothalamus. Because of
this, the chanting of mantras has been used as an adjunctive therapy against
an array of conditions, including HIV infection, autoimmune diseases,
arthritis, memory loss, and allergies.

BRAIN UNIFICATION

Another important effect of the chanting of mantras is the unification of the brain. As you probably know, the left and right hemispheres of the brain are notably independent. Because of this, a person with damage to just one side of the brain can sometimes recover full function by retraining the undamaged side of the brain.

Even various areas of each hemisphere have independent functions. For example, the left hemisphere of the brain contains two important areas that have very different linguistic functions. One area is Broca's area, which is in the lower left frontal area. Broca's area governs the structures of language, such as grammar. If Broca's area is damaged, a person can speak understandably but will have extremely poor sentence structure and grammar. Another related area is Wernicke's area, which is farther back in the left hemisphere's temporal lobe. Wernicke's area enables people to express meaningful thoughts. If this area is damaged, people will speak grammatically but will simply string together meaningless, inappropriate phrases. To be fluent in speech, both Broca's area and Wernicke's area must function in full coordination and communication. The very best way to achieve this coordination is just by speaking meaningful, grammatical phrases. Furthermore, the repetition of meaningful, grammatical phrases heightens this ability.

But there are even more differences between the two hemispheres of the brain than between different areas in the same hemisphere. The right hemisphere is active when you sing, rhyme, make vowel sounds, create metaphors, and speak with emotion. The left hemisphere is relatively more involved with nonemotional statements, proper word usage, grammar, logic, and consonant sounds. The two hemispheres are connected primarily by a band of nerves called the corpus callosum, and secondarily by the limbic system and hypothalamus. These structures connect emotion to logic, vowels to consonants, and grammar to metaphor.

The best way to activate and connect the two hemispheres is through repetitive use of particular phrases. When repetitive phrasing is combined with breath and patterned movement, the two sides of the brain are stimulated to function in optimal concert. This harmonious function of the brain creates the best healing environment through the triad of mind, body, and spirit. The endocrine system is balanced, the nervous system is energized, and circulation is stimulated.

ETHEREAL ENERGY FLOW

Another effect of chanting mantras is the stimulation of energy flow through the nadis. The human body has 72,000 nadis, nonphysical energy channels analogous to nerves. Prana travels through these nadis and energizes the entire system, particularly the chakras. The three central nadis are the *ida* and *pingala,* which are on each side of the spine, and the *shushmana,* which runs up the center of the spine to the head.

When you recite vibratory mantras, they vibrate the topmost part of the central channel, the shushmana. It also inhibits the flow of thoughts, which can interfere with energy flow in the shushmana.

To most effectively stimulate the shushmana, it is important to have the proper mental attitude, which reduces thoughts that interfere with the energy flow. The proper attitude is one of nonattachment and devotion, or *bhakti.* To further heighten energy flow, one must also achieve the condition of *shakti,* which is the power that is created by the discipline of repetition. The flow of energy through the nadis is also greatly increased by proper breath, posture, and movement.

QUIETING THE INNER DIALOGUE

Yet another advantage of chanting mantras is that they help to quiet the inner dialogue, the constant chatter that goes on in the mind. Unfortunately, this chatter is often harmful. It frequently consists of a critical internal voice—created as a survival mechanism—that warns us about possible threats. It's good to know about threats, but we generally take this action too far, and create constant, low-level anxiety for ourselves. When the inner dialogue becomes too negative and fearful, it activates the fight-or-flight, sympathetic branch of the nervous system. When this occurs, it drains energy from the rest-and-repair, parasympathetic branch. This creates the stress hormones that lower immunity and interfere with cognitive function.

Furthermore, the inner dialogue distances us from the moment-to-moment experience of reality. It clutters our brains with worry and trivia, and keeps us from intimate contact with the small moments that create our lives and the magic that so often lies behind these moments.

Another problem with the internal dialogue is that it tends to split the psyche in two. Our optimistic self argues with our pessimistic self, our intuition fights our logic, and our generous side jousts with our selfishness. At worst, we're reduced to schizoid half-beings, bereft of wholeness. By temporarily halting these constant battles of self-versus-self, the chanting of mantras endows us with the single-mindedness that is needed for a life of passion, commitment, and peace.

REPLICATION OF DNA

The final important action of the chanting of mantras, or primordial sounds, is simultaneously quite scientific and quite esoteric. This action is the ability of sound to heighten the proper replication of DNA.

DNA (or deoxyribonucleic acid) carries the essential information of life. DNA, found in the nucleus of every living cell on earth, is the complex combination of just four chemicals, composed in strands. These four chemicals, in their multitude of combinations, carry the information that allows cells to produce replicas of themselves. This replication is essential, of course, since each cell has only a short life, far shorter than the life of the entire organism. Cells in the mouth, for example, are replaced every few days, and all the cells in the brain are replaced every year. This replacement is effective, though, only when the cell has the proper DNA information to create a perfect replica.

Unfortunately, DNA often becomes damaged, resulting in imperfect replicas. This can, among other things, contribute to the process of aging. It can also allow a healthy cell to be reborn as a malignant cell. Therefore, it is vitally important to protect DNA. One way to do this is simply to engage in a healthy lifestyle, which offers the DNA a maximum of nutritional building blocks, and a minimum of toxic assaults. Another way is to nurture the DNA with universal, primordial vibrations, or sounds—and this is where our examination of DNA becomes relatively more esoteric.

In *Quantum Healing*, Deepak Chopra, M.D., states, "You may not think that you can 'talk' to your DNA, but in fact you do it continually." Dr. Chopra notes that the language with which we speak to our own DNA consists of primordial sound. Disease can occur, Dr. Chopra believes, when there is a communication breakdown in the circle of body, mind, and DNA. "To repair the break," he writes, "a specific signal needs to be inserted back into the circle— a primordial sound. In this way, a vibration is used to cure a vibration."

"If you were enlightened," Dr. Chopra maintains, "you would be able to hear the vibration that is your own signature; for instance, you could 'hear' your own DNA as a specific frequency vibrating in your awareness. Likewise, each neuropeptide would grow out of a sound, as would every other chemical. Starting with DNA, the whole body unfolds into many levels, and at each one . . . the sequence of sound comes first. Therefore, putting a primordial sound back into the body is like reminding it what station it should be tuned into."

Dr. Gurucharan Singh makes a similar statement, in a somewhat different way. "Each complete Shabd," he notes, "adds an inheritance, a spiritual DNA, that establishes your identity and lineage with Infinity—the unknowable unknown, itself."

These are the physical effects of the Shabd Guru. But they are not the only effects. The Shabd Guru does not merely change the body. After all, words, quite obviously, also communicate ideas. And ideas can heal.

The following mantras will help you heal. They have mystical powers. Most of them are ancient mantras that contain not only healing sounds, but healing ideas. I have used them in my medical practice, and in my own life, for many years.

These powerful mantras belong to the ages. And now they will belong, also, to you.

Mantras

Ong Namo, Guru Dev Namo

This mantra is always the first that is chanted during a session of kundalini yoga or meditation, and is therefore referred to as the Tuning In to your Higher Self Mantra. The literal meaning is, "I bow before my highest consciousness." The mantra should be chanted loudly, from the back of the nasal cavity and from the throat. As a rule, it is chanted in prayer pose, with the hands near the heart, palms together, and the knuckles of the thumbs pressed against the breastbone.

Guru Guru Wahe Guru Guru Ram Das Guru

This mantra is referred to as the Miracle Mantra, because it has served as a primary component in many healing miracles. Its physical effect is to evoke deep relaxation, which is the ideal physiological state for healing. Its literal meaning is as follows: *Guru* means "divine wisdom," or teacher. *Wahe guru* refers to the infinite wisdom of God. *Ram* means God. *Das* means service. Thus, the phrase literally means, "Divine wisdom, infinite wisdom, service of God." Ram Das is also the name of a person, a spiritual leader of the sixteenth century, who built the Golden Temple. The great Guru Ram Das was noted for his healing powers, compassion, and humility.

The feeling produced by this mantra is a sensation of protection and healing, brought about by God being with you.

A close friend of mine, named Linda, used this mantra to help achieve a healing miracle with her son. The boy was gravely ill, and was not expected to live through the night, but my friend played a tape recording of this mantra all night long in his hospital room, while meditating upon the mantra, and by the next morning the child had recovered, astonishing the hospital's doctors, nurses, and staff.

Om

This mantra is considered by some to be the most basic sound of the universe. It is composed of the three sounds *ah, oh,* and *m,* and refers, in the Hindu tradition, to the trinity of creation, preservation, and destruction. There is a passive element to this mantra that may not be appropriate for active Westerners, who may be better served by the mantra Ong. Both *om* and *ong* have strong vibratory effects. While *om* refers to the force of creation, *ong* refers to the Creator, who is the Doer of all action.

Raa Maa Daa Saa Saa Say So Hung

This powerful mantra is the Mantra for Healing Self and Others. Filled with vibratory vowels and primordial sounds, it has an energizing effect upon the neurological and endocrine systems. The literal translation is as follows: *Raa* means sun; *Maa* means moon; *Daa* means earth; *Saa* means totality of experience; *So* means personal sense of identity; and *Hung* means the Infinite vibration.

When these words are combined, the essential meaning is, "I am thou." Another meaning is, "The service of God is within me."

If you wish to heal yourself with this mantra, imagine a glowing green light around you as you meditate. To heal others, imagine that the light is around them.

See the final chapter for the full Medical Meditation to Heal Self and Others, which includes the posture for this meditation.

Sa Ta Na Ma

This mantra, which is used in the important Kirtan Kriya, is called the Panch Shabd, or Primal Sound Mantra, because it consists of the five primal sounds: *S, T, N, M,* and *ah.* The literal meaning is as follows: *Sa* means birth (or infinity); *Ta* means life; *Na* means death; and *Ma* means rebirth. Thus, the mantra describes the eternal circle of life: birth, life, death, rebirth.

The physical benefits of the mantra are:

- *Sa* evokes a sense of emotion and expansiveness.
- *Ta* creates a feeling of transformation and strength.
- *Na* stimulates a sense of universal love.
- *Ma* evokes the quality of communicativeness.

One powerful way to use this mantra is to chant it for two minutes in your normal voice, which I call the voice of action. Then whisper it for two minutes, in the voice of the lover. For the next three minutes, chant silently, in the divine language. Then reverse the order, for a total of eleven minutes of chanting. (Another description of these three modes of speech is that they are, respectively, the voice of the body, the mind, and the spirit.)

Sat Nam

This is a Bij Mantra, or Seed Mantra. It is the most widely used mantra in the practice of kundalini yoga. *Sat* means truth, and *Nam* means identity. Thus, the phrase means, "Truth is my identity." It also means, "The essence of God is within me." The mantra has a strong balancing effect, and is believed to awaken the soul. It is often used as a greeting or salutation. Like Sa Ta Na Ma, it is composed of the five primal sounds. Sat may be chanted or thought on the inhale, while Nam is usually chanted or thought on the exhale.

Wahe Guru

This simple mantra is the Guru Mantra, or Mantra of Ecstasy. It is pronounced, "Wah-hay Gu-roó." The Wahe Guru mantra is the mantra of the *ajna,* or third eye. From the Western perspective, therefore, it is the mantra that most effectively stimulates the pituitary gland. The sound *wah* is considered to be the sound of Aquarius; it is the sound that is produced when water is poured out of a narrow opening in a bottle, as air enters.

The sound *guru* can either be extended, or said quickly. *Wah,* however, should always be said quickly. The most important sound in the mantra is *he*—pronounced "hay." It means, "I have gained."

When you say this mantra, focus upon the joy that you have achieved through knowledge and experience, and particularly upon the ecstasy that you have received by experiencing the nature of the Infinite, or divine.

A variation of this mantra is Wahe Guru, Wahe Guru, Wahe Guru, Wahe Jio (pronounced "gee-o"). *Jio* is an affectionate term for the soul. This mantra means, "O my soul, when I experience the indescribable wisdom of God, I am in ecstasy."

Following are other mantras that were not derived from the tradition of the Shabd Guru. Most are in English. Therefore, they do not necessarily contain the particular combinations of sounds that have specific physiological effects upon the brain and endocrine system. Nonetheless, these mantras, or prayers, are important components of various great religions, and are therefore rich in meaning and spiritual power. You can gain some of the vibratory benefits of these mantras, however, by elongating their vowel sounds. For example, the Hebrew word *shalom,* which is a powerful mantra meaning peace, ends in the primal sound *om,* which can be accented and elongated to increase its vibratory effects.

Hail Mary, full of grace, the Lord is with thee. Blessed art thou among women, and blessed is the fruit of thy womb, Jesus. Holy Mary, mother of God, pray for us sinners, now and at the hour of our death. Amen.

The familiar Hail Mary celebrates the announcement by the angel Gabriel of the personification of God on earth. It is an important part of the liturgy of the Catholic Church. In the Catholic faith, it is chanted repeatedly, as part of the rosary. It has been used during innumerable instances of healing miracles and spiritual breakthroughs. It is traditionally recited during the final moments of a person's life, not only for its intrinsic power but also to help return the dying person to the state of union with God that he or she has experienced many times before, during the recitation of the rosary.

Shalom

This is one of the oldest religious mantras. It is a Hebrew word meaning peace, which is often used casually as a salutation. Pronounced "shaw-loam," it ends with the primordial sound *om*. This sound may be elongated, in order to derive vibratory benefit.

The Lord Is My Shepherd

This phrase is the beginning of the Twenty-third Psalm, one of the most beautiful and powerful passages in the Bible. The entire psalm, as well as this phrase, is a favorite of the Christian Church. It celebrates the protective power of God, and is excellent at evoking the feeling that even in peril, a person is still sheltered by the benign force of universal preservation: "Yea, though I walk through the valley of the shadow of death, I will fear no evil, for Thou art with me."

God and Me, Me and God Are One

This nonsectarian mantra refers to the universality of divinity. It reminds people that to find God, they need look no further than within. Finding divinity in oneself is the ultimate empowerment.

Healthy Am I, Happy Am I, Holy Am I

Repetition of this nonsectarian mantra teaches a person that health, happiness, and holiness are inseparable, and are each equal reflections of the nature of God. I have seen this mantra employed very favorably in several medical outcomes.

Hear O Israel, the Lord Our God, the Lord Is One

This is the translation of the Hebrew prayer Shama Yesroael ("Hear O Israel"). When sung freely in the original Hebrew, it gives the singer the feeling that God is near.

CHAPTER SEVEN

Mental Focus

The Mind-Power Effect

The mind—consisting of thoughts in the brain—can heal.

It does so primarily through the phenomenon of psychoneuro-immunology. Thoughts trigger responses by the hypothalamus and pituitary, similar to the way that physical actions, such as sound vibrations, trigger responses of the hypothalamus and pituitary. It's quite reasonable that thoughts can trigger these actions, since the hypothalamus and pituitary act as links between the mind and body. For example, positive, calming thoughts can heighten immunity, by causing the nervous system to shift into its healing, rest-and-repair branch (the parasympathetic branch).

In addition, mind-power healing can also occur in ways that don't directly involve the immune system. For example, calming thoughts can help solve the condition of irregular heartbeat, which is not related to immune system problems.

The mind-power effect upon healing is so profound that it heals many physical problems by itself, with no further therapy. Also, it helps solve other problems when used as an adjunctive therapy. The mind-power effect boosts the healing power of effective medicines by an estimated 30 percent, when patients believe the medicine they are taking will help them. It also often creates a healing effect with an ineffective medication, through the well-known placebo effect. If your mind is burdened by negativity, though, you may suffer a negative mind-power effect. Studies show that when people believe their medications won't help, or might even be harmful, they are far less likely to gain benefit from the medications.

Some people have very highly developed abilities of mind-power healing. In one case at the University of Arkansas College of Medicine, a woman demonstrated the ability to alter her immune response at will. The woman could change her skin test for the chicken pox virus, varicella zoster, just by thinking specific thoughts. When she focused on sending healing energy to her body, she could change her viral blood test from positive to negative. By willing the virus to return, she could then change her blood test response from negative to positive.

Having this degree of mind-power healing is relatively uncommon in the general population. However, a heightened degree of this ability appears to be common among the small subpopulation of advanced meditators. Furthermore, having a moderate amount of mind-power healing ability is quite common. In fact, the majority of people have at least some degree of mind-power healing ability. This degree can be increased, with a moderate amount of effort.

One of the most practical ways to measure the effectiveness of the mind-power effect in large population groups is to analyze health data on people with strong, positive religious feelings, who frequently pray. Although not all religious people have fundamentally positive mental outlooks, religious faith is considered to be generally indicative of a positive outlook and an overriding sense of personal security. Furthermore, prayer almost always evokes a positive outlook. Prayer, of course, is a form of meditation, and causes most of the same helpful, physiological reactions that are created by other forms of meditation.

Following is a sample of the many studies that have been done on the health of people with strong religious beliefs.

- In a long-term study of mortality, 5.4 percent of churchgoers died, compared to 17.3 percent of nonchurchgoers.
- In a study of disability among the elderly due to illness or injury, lack of religious faith was an even stronger predictor of disability than an unhealthy lifestyle.
- A study of high blood pressure found that religious people were 40 percent less likely to have diastolic hypertension than nonreligious people.
- In a study of coronary heart disease, religious men suffered 20 percent less incidence of the disease than nonreligious men.

- A study of immunity found that nonreligious people had twice as much of a protein that indicates immune weakness as did religious people. (The protein was interleukin-6.)
- In a study of cancer patients, patients who received a program of spiritual and religious counseling lived approximately twice as long after diagnosis as patients who did not.

Of course, religious people often have healthier lifestyles than nonreligious people, and this may be a factor in their superior health. However, the researchers in many of these studies took that factor into account, and tried to match lifestyle habits of religious and nonreligious people.

Other studies and experiments also reveal the potency of the mind-power effect. Some of the most fascinating experiments were done on simple organisms, such as bacteria and yeast, that are unable to think, thus ruling out any psychosomatic factors.

In one experiment, human subjects tried to slow down growth of yeast, just by focusing their mental power on the task. Of 194 dishes of yeast, growth was successfully slowed in 151. This experiment was replicated sixteen times, with similar results in all sixteen trials. In addition, subjects (none of whom had any special healing abilities) were also able to speed up yeast growth. Furthermore, subjects were able to alter the growth of yeast from a distance of sixteen miles away, illustrating a fundamental principle of the mind-power effect: It transcends space. In many other experiments, the mind-power effect was just as strong from a distance as it was during close contact.

In one particularly astonishing series of experiments, conducted at Princeton University, the mind-power effect even seemed to influence an inanimate object—a machine. In this series of 256,000 trials, conducted over several years, subjects tried to influence a computer-like machine that generated random numbers. The database derived from these trials was the largest of its kind that has ever been developed. The goal of the subjects was to make the machine generate distinct patterns of numbers, instead of random numbers. The success achieved was considered not just statistically significant, but overwhelming. People did, indeed, appear to be capable of influencing the machine.

Interestingly, they were best able to influence the machine after they had achieved a sense of empathetic bonding with it, similar to the feeling that some people have for their automobiles. Even more interesting was the fact that people could influence the machine by applying the mind-power effect before the machine actually began to operate.

Most fascinating of all, subjects could influence the machine after it had already run. This outcome contradicts conventional thought, of course, because almost all people believe that once an event has occurred, nothing can change it—and certainly not mind-power intervention from the future. Nonetheless, this research was properly conducted, and consisted of large numbers of independent trials. Therefore, the outcome of this particular experiment can only be considered mysterious—or perhaps a glimpse into the unknowable. In any case, it does appear to suggest that the mind-power effect may not be governed by the ordinary constraints of time, just as it is not limited by the ordinary constraints of space.

The phenomenon of mind-power healing has also been successfully applied to animals. In one prominent study, conducted by Dr. Bernard Grad of McGill University, an accomplished mental healer was able to significantly speed healing of laboratory animals by using the mind-power effect.

In a related study, the same healer, using only his mental powers, was able to protect laboratory animals from developing goiters after the animals had been injected with a goiter-producing drug. Other animals were also given the drug, but were not subjected to the mind-power effect. Virtually all of these animals did develop goiters.

Achieving results with the mind-power effect, however, does not require an accomplished healer. Nor does it even require a strong, intentional focus. For example, in one experiment, laboratory animal handlers were told that some animals had been given high dosages of a malaria microorganism, while other animals had been given low dosages. In fact, though, all the animals had been given identical dosages. Nonetheless, the animals that the handlers thought had been given high, disease-causing dosages fared much worse than the others.

Of course, mind-power experiments have also been performed with human subjects. The most interesting experiments were those in which the mind-power healers focused upon other people, because this ruled out the possibility of psychosomatic self-healing. In one famous study, conducted by cardiologist Randolph Byrd at San Francisco General Hospital, prayer was used to influence the medical outcomes of heart disease patients. Prayer, of course, is by far the most common type of mind-power healing used in contemporary cultures. In Dr. Byrd's study, which consisted of 393 patients, approximately half the patients were prayed for by other people, without the patients knowing that this was occurring. The patients who were prayed for did significantly better than the others: they were five times less likely to require antibiotics, and three times less likely to develop pulmonary edema. None of the patients who were prayed for required an artificial breathing apparatus, but twelve who were not prayed for did. In addition, somewhat fewer of the patients who were prayed for died.

Of course, many people would ascribe these results to the intervention of God. This may well be accurate. However, all we know with certainty is that the mind-power effect was applied, and that it did apparently activate a healing source of an unknown origin.

Dr. Byrd's study is just one of many that have been conducted on the subject of intentional influence upon human beings and other living organisms using the mind-power effect. As Larry Dossey, M.D., points out in his eloquent book *Healing Words,* these studies generally indicate that thought can influence the physical condition of human beings, animals, plants, cells, and microorganisms. Dr. Dossey notes that 131 controlled trials have been conducted, and that 77 demonstrated statistically significant, positive results. Of these 77 studies, 56 yielded outcomes in which the possibility that the results were due to chance was less than 1 out of 100. Another 21 of the 77 studies yielded outcomes in which the possibility that the results were due to chance was between 2 and 5 out of 100.

Other recent studies also strongly indicate the medical efficacy of mind-power healing, including prayer. Among the studies are the following:

- A study by Elisabeth Targ, M.D., of forty AIDS patients tested the efficacy of prayer performed on behalf of the patients by others, who were not in proximity to the patients. The patients did not know whether they were in the group being prayed for or in a control group. The study concluded, "Patients who received treatment [prayer] had a statistically significant more benign course than control patients." They experienced notably fewer complications, required less medical intervention, and reported a more positive mental outlook. The patients were examined according to twenty-seven different baseline measures. Dr. Targ later commented, "Every way we sliced this pie, the treatment group was less ill."

Dr. Targ has recently completed another research project involving breast cancer patients. In this study women are utilizing meditation and prayer as part of a broad-based integrative program (which includes art therapy, group discussion, and nutrition). Moreover, Dr. Targ has begun a follow-up study on distant healing and AIDS, and will also soon be doing a study on the healing effects of the Sat Nam Rasayan, a Medical Meditation distant healing technique. This study will involve patients with diabetes.

- A study by Bentwich and Kreitler examined patients recovering from hernia surgery, in regard to mind-power effects that were applied to their recoveries. The patients were divided into three groups; one group received a single prayer from a distance, another group listened to a healing imagery tape, and the third (control) group received no extra intervention. The group that had been prayed for fared best. They experienced better outcomes on wound healing, fever rates, care satisfaction, and general well-being.

- In a study by William Braud, M.D., subjects demonstrated a statistically significant ability to protect their own extracted blood, placed in test tubes, from damage. The blood was exposed to a contaminant that causes blood cells to die. At the same time the blood was exposed, the subjects were directed to protect their blood with mental energy. Nine of 32 subjects were able to inhibit damage to their blood samples. The probability of this happening by chance is approximately 1 in 50,000.

Dr. Larry Dossey has examined many of the studies on prayer, to try to determine what type of mind-power influence was most effective. What he has discovered goes against the grain of conventional wisdom. Most people presume that the best way to achieve a particular outcome is to focus directly upon it. This includes praying for a specific outcome. However, Dr. Dossey found that people achieved their most satisfying results when they did not actively yearn for, or pray for, a specific outcome, but instead simply let go, and got in touch with their highest, most spiritually evolved selves. For example, Dr. Dossey found that people who had achieved healing miracles, against all odds, usually had not been obsessed with healing. "One of their chief characteristics," Dr. Dossey writes, "is that they do not determinedly want healing; they are not desperate for a miracle to occur. . . . They have a quality of acceptance and gratitude, as if things are quite all right in spite of the presence of the disease. Thus the paradox: Those who do not demand healing are the ones who frequently seem to receive it."

Dr. Dossey wisely notes, "Attempting to use only the consciously aware part of the mind is like trying to shoot an arrow by pushing it forward from the bow string. Everyone knows it's best to pull the string back and let the power of the bow do the work. In many situations, one has to let go, in the realization that there are simply some things one cannot make happen."

This sort of surrender, however, is not the same thing as just giving up. With surrender, there is an expectation that whatever happens will be acceptable. When you give up, though, you tend to expect the worst, and dread it.

Because of the ironic power of surrender, one of the most potent forms of the mind-power effect is the type of prayer called nondirected prayer. In nondirected prayer, there is no request for a specific outcome. Instead, the person who prays focuses on the feeling that things happen for the best, and focuses upon his or her desire to see events unfold naturally, according to the benign flow of the universe.

Nondirected prayer, as well as other forms of prayer, have been scientifically studied for many years by an Oregon scientific association called Spindrift. In one interesting experiment conducted by the Spindrift organization, subjects used nondirected prayer as well as directed prayer (in which they asked for a specific outcome). Their prayers were directed at a nonthinking organism—a culture of bacteria—to avoid the possibility of a psychosomatic response. When the directed prayer was applied, no results were achieved. Nondirected prayer, however, achieved positive results of more robust, longer-lived colonies of bacteria.

The Spindrift organization conducted many other experiments on nondirected prayer, and found that nondirected prayer evoked powerful and predictable results in a statistically significant number of cases. Based upon these experiments, the Spindrift organization concluded that when nondirected prayer was applied, the outcome tended to be whatever was best for the organism that was being prayed for. For example, in one experiment involving germinating beans, some of the beans were oversoaked with water, and some were undersoaked. When all of the beans were prayed for in a nondirected manner, those that had been oversoaked began to eliminate water, and those that had been undersoaked began to absorb water. This did not occur in a control group of beans.

The Spindrift organization did conclude, however, that nondirected prayer is not inherently superior for all people. Some people simply feel more comfortable with directed prayer. For each individual, the best type of prayer is the one that feels most comfortable. Personally, I employ both types of prayer virtually every morning. First, I pray for the well-being of my children and wife, for the health of my patients, and for progress in the work I am trying to accomplish. Then I drift into a nondirected state of higher consciousness, meditate on the perfection of the universe, and ask for the right thing to happen. For me, this is the most fulfilling way to manifest the mind-power effect, and to get in touch with my highest self.

During either nondirected prayer or directed prayer, however, there is one element that appears to significantly empower the prayer: love. Love makes the mind-power effect even more powerful, and it also appears to have a healing effect of its own, even in the absence of meditation.

The intrinsic healing power of love was demonstrated in a recent experiment at the Harvard Medical School. A group of subjects was shown a documentary film of Mother Theresa showering kindness upon vulnerable people. The film was intended to evoke feelings of altruism, generosity, and love among those who viewed it. Researchers then measured a key component of the subjects' immune systems (immunoglobulin-A), and compared it to measurements that had been taken before the subjects had seen the film. In a statistically significant number of subjects, the immune system marker had risen, indicating increased immunity. This occurred even among subjects who considered Mother Theresa to be too religious.

The Harvard researchers then tried a similar experiment without the film. Instead of showing subjects the film, the researchers asked them to focus upon people they loved, or times when they felt loved. Again, their immune systems showed heightened power. Both of these experiments, as you probably noticed, did not actively involve the mind-power effect. The power of love, alone, was the only mental force that was applied.

An interesting example of the strengthening influence of love upon the mind-power effect comes from the series of Princeton studies in which people tried to influence a machine. The machine, as you may recall, issued random numbers, while the subjects in the experiment tried to make the machine issue orderly patterns of numbers. This experiment involved not only individuals, but also pairs of people. Some of the pairs were couples who were in love. Among all subjects, those who were most capable of influencing the machine were the couples who were in love.

Love appears to be a factor not only in mind-power healing, but also in other esoteric mental powers that are still shrouded in mystery, such as telepathy, the ability to transmit thoughts mentally. Researcher F. W. H. Myers, who has conducted numerous scientific studies of telepathy, has concluded that love, more than any other psychological factor, is the most powerful conduit for telepathy. He has stated, "Love is a kind of exalted but unspecialized telepathy—the simplest and most universal expression of the mutual gravitation, or kinship of spirits, which is the foundation for the telepathic law." Love, Myers believes, accounts for the relatively commonplace occurrence of someone knowing that a loved one is hurt, or has died, before the information actually reaches them.

It is also widely believed that love is the primary force that makes it possible for one person to help heal another person from a distance, using the mind-power effect. This phenomenon, generally referred to as distant healing, has been documented by a number of researchers, including Dr. Randolph Byrd. However, even the term distant healing is actually a misnomer, according to Dr. Larry Dossey, the world's most prominent author on the subject of the power of prayer. Dr. Dossey states, "There is no such thing as distant healing, because there is no distance separating people that must be overcome. This means that healing of another is in some sense self-healing, for the spatial distinctions between 'self' and 'other' are not fundamental. . . . Empathy, compassion, and love seem to form a literal bond—a resonance, or glue—between living things."

I have experienced this rare and exquisite bond myself, as a doctor of medicine who helps to heal, and as a human being who helps to heal. I wish words could fully communicate the feeling this bond creates, but they cannot. Like other of life's most precious experiences, this feeling can't be described, but only felt.

Medical Meditation will help bring you closer to your highest self, closer to perfect health, and closer even to love. When you do experience this feeling, you will more completely comprehend these wise words by the great Dr. Carl Jung: "Man can try to name love, showering upon it all the names at his command, and he will still involve himself in endless self-deceptions. If he possesses a grain of wisdom, he will lay down his arms and name the unknown by the more unknown . . . by the name of God."

As you begin to practice Medical Meditation, you will notice that the focus of concentration is often the tip of the nose. This stimulates the pituitary gland because the optic nerves run right next to the gland, and the stretch produced by the eye focus tonifies the pituitary. Concentrating at the third eye, which is found at the root of the nose between the eyebrows, also stimulates the pituitary gland. Focusing on the top of the head has a similar effect on the pineal gland. As you progress in your capacity to meditate, you will notice how much more mindful you are of the sounds you create and the vibrations generated by these sounds in your skull. These vibrations act as a brain massage and orchestrate the mind-power effect I discussed in this chapter. You can also focus on the meaning of the mantra. This will help you develop a more refined healing ability.

The most effective focus, however, is when you color your positive and loving healing intention with the power of prana. By combining this pure vibration with breath work, you can project your energy to transcend time and space, thereby filling the void of separation that often is mistakenly felt to exist between yourself and others. Entering the zone of the meditative mind, you discover the power to increase the caliber of your healing talent and, if you wish, direct this light not only to yourself but someone else as well.

Two Medical Meditation techniques found in the final chapter will help you develop and utilize the highest powers of your mind—Medical Meditation to Transfer Healing Energy (see page 271), and Medical Meditation to Heal Self and Others (see page 272). It is often said that the highest state of spiritual living is selfless service, or *seva*—the capacity to give to others without thought of reward. As you practice these Medical Meditations to help others, you may well find that seva leads to a true and lasting happiness.

CHAPTER EIGHT

Sadhana

Combining the Elements of
Healing in Daily Practice

The desert wakes in the night and sleeps in the day. When the foothills of the Catalina Mountains behind my house break free from the fiery daylight, nocturnal animals awaken and desert plants open themselves up for a nightly drink of dew. But the oasis of human life that people have created within this desert operates on the opposite schedule, with imported patio plants opening to the sun and closing to the dark.

At each cusp between light and dark, though, both desert and domestic life stir and buzz, whether preparing to awaken or to sleep. These junctions hold great energy, even though this energy is often caught in the blurry midworld between action and slumber.

If this energy can be tapped—and I believe it can—great power can be captured. The modern mystic Carlos Castaneda called the twilight of late evening and early morning the crack between the two worlds, and he often tried to slip through this crack, into the world of his highest self.

Early each morning I, too, try to slip away from the material and mundane, because I have found that the rare chronobiological power of this magical time can carry me through the rest of the day feeling strong, resilient, and open.

On one recent early summer day, we began our usual routine of early morning prayer, yoga, and meditation. At first, in the dark of earliest day, it was hard, and I longed for the softness of bed. But as the sun grew strong, so did I, and the most difficult yoga positions suddenly became easy, just as a hard ball game gets easy once you slide into its flow. Soon, everything felt so effortless and right that it seemed as if my breaths were breathing me, instead of the other way around. I could see that Kirti felt the same, and it gave us a special closeness.

After meditating, I strolled onto our red tile patio and began to watch a flower unfold. I once thought of this as an impossibly slow process—something to observe only through time-lapse film—but I've found that with a modicum of patience and personal power I can make this unfolding seem fast and exciting. It is especially easy with very sun-sensitive flowers, such as the purple morning glory I was watching on this day. With new sun on its petals, the morning glory practically sprang to life. It came awake as quickly, and at the same time, as the hummingbirds, rabbits, and squirrels around our house, to become, with them, part of the living mosaic of our domestic oasis.

The most obvious function of the awakened flower, of course, was simply to be beautiful—to attract with color the insects and birds that propagate its life from summer to summer. But beneath this placid function was a roiling, invisible whirl of biological action: nutrient absorption, photosynthesis, and the restless journey of roots and stems. There was nothing passive about the morning glory. It was infinitely active, as are all living things, including all human beings. It is through this activity—and only through this activity—that we can become our highest selves.

In his wise book *Sadhana: The Realization of Life,* Nobel Prize–winning poet Rabindranath Tagore notes, "There are many who imagine action to be opposed to freedom. They think that activity, being in the material plane, is a restriction of the free spirit of the soul. But we must remember: The soul finds its freedom in action." The texts of the Upanishads say the same thing: "In the midst of activity alone wilt thou desire to live a hundred years."

The ancient yoga masters, who first created the advanced meditations that I have adapted as Medical Meditations, felt exactly the same way. They thought that no power, nor any healing, could come without effort. I agree with this wholeheartedly. There can be no healing without hard work. And there can be no fullness of life without great effort.

And so, after I had watched the flower unfold and focused on its endless activity, I was excited for the day to continue. I went inside, dressed, and prepared to meet a patient.

* * *

My patient was late. She dragged herself into the office with lidded eyes, clutching coffee, and slumped into a chair. I felt as if I had seen her before, and in a way, I had. She was the single most typical patient that enters any doctor's office: a person in midlife with a chronic, mild physical ailment that's suddenly somewhat worse than usual. In addition to their focal-point problem, these patients usually have a similar set of generic symptoms: low energy, insomnia, malaise, and aches and pains. This type of patient is generally considered to account for approximately 33 percent of all doctor visits.

For many years, doctors dismissed these patients as hypochondriacs, prescribed for them as harmless a palliative as possible, and sent them away. Then, during the height of the Prozac Revolution, it was in vogue to ascribe this predictable stew of symptoms to clinical depression, and to bombard the patient with serotonin-enhancing drugs. More recently, it's become clinically correct to categorize these people as the worried well, and to nod sympathetically, establish rapport, and then urge them gently out the door.

This woman, Jane, a forty-two-year-old Tucson yarn-shop owner who'd heard about my work with chronic pain, began to tell me about mild symptoms of fibromyalgia that she had been experiencing. She also started describing the generic symptoms—insomnia, malaise—and pointing out the places where her muscles hurt. And then she just ran out of gas and dropped the whole subject.

"It's not all *that* bad," Jane said. "I just thought maybe . . ."

I stayed quiet, because I felt she was headed toward the truth, and I'm always amazed at how well talk hides truth.

She sighed from deep in her belly. "I'm just a garden-variety neurotic," she blurted. "*That's* what I need treatment for. In my opinion."

"Can't help you," I said.

Jane gave me a funny look.

"According to the medical profession," I said, "there is no longer a mental condition called neurosis. It's gone! They took it out of the *Diagnostic and Statistical Manual,* the bible of mental diagnoses. Doctors can't even bill insurance companies for it anymore."

"It's gone?" she asked incredulously.

"You're cured," I said, smiling. But she wasn't cured. She just wasn't neurotic.

Her blank look told me that she was dumbfounded. For most of her adult life, she had probably placed her identity inside the convenient box called "neurotic." As for millions of other people, this medical label had been her shield and her sword. Of course she couldn't be happy—she was neurotic. Of course she couldn't give herself over to complete love—she was neurotic. Of course she couldn't be healthy, or energetic, or success-ful. Who could, with her . . . mental illness?

Jane had learned to see herself primarily in terms of the wounds inflicted upon her by life. She was all wrapped up in what Caroline Myss, Ph.D., calls woundology. She used her wound to connect to other wounded people, to reach for help, and to find meaning in a life that had lost sense. However, as Dr. Myss says, "Healing means getting over pain, not 'market-ing' it."

In fairness to my patient, though, the medical profession had perpetu-ated this woundology—and profited from it. But now it was time to put an end to it.

She came out of her bewilderment and asked, "Well, if I'm not neu-rotic, what is wrong with me?"

"Exactly the things you said. Muscle pains. Insomnia. Malaise. Low energy."

"But I'm not neurotic?" She was having a hard time getting used to the idea.

"You're the same person you were when you walked in. Descriptions change. Language changes. But you're still you."

"What's causing all my problems, then?"

"I want to be honest with you, and whenever you're honest, there's never an easy answer to a hard question. So I can't just say it's low sero-tonin, or it's hypothyroidism, or it's a low-grade candida infection—even though all of those factors may be present. Sometimes it's a lot smarter to think less about the cause and more about the cure. I know conventional medicine says you can't cure anything without knowing the cause, but that's just not always true. It sounds scientific, but it's actually simplistic. Causes are often so multifactored, and so interwoven, that they're just a big, impenetrable mystery. Whenever I run into that, I try to forget about illness, and focus on health. Let me tell you about one of the best things you can possibly do for your health. It's Medical Meditation, and I think it will solve a number of your problems, all at once."

"I like meditation," Jane said. "It's pleasant."

"It is pleasant. But it's hard, too. Medical Meditation requires a lot of activity."

She looked uneasy. That was good. She was beginning to understand. She was in for the challenge of her life.

How to Do Basic Meditation

Meditating is easy to learn. Living a meditative lifestyle is harder. Let's start with the easy part. Here's how to meditate. To be ready, all you need are comfort, quiet, a meditative tool (such as a mantra), and a meditative attitude.

- Go to a private place by yourself, or with another meditator, where you won't be interrupted.
- Allow ten to twenty minutes for meditation, and stick with it. You can look at your watch on occasion, but don't set an alarm, because it might startle you and ruin your relaxation.
- Sit down on a comfortable mat, cushion, or chair, and try to relax every muscle in your body, from bottom to top. Close your eyes, and breathe deeply.
- To help stop your internal dialogue, and help calm down, silently repeat a word or mantra. It can be religious, or philosophical, as long as it makes you feel good. When thoughts intrude, just say, "Oh, well," to yourself, and start over.
- Adopt a calm, passive attitude—a neutral mind, in which you don't judge yourself or others.
- After you finish, sit quietly for a couple of minutes, and try to carry your calm meditative attitude into your daily activities.

Many of my patients say, "I've tried to meditate but gave up because of all the thoughts going through my mind." Don't let this stop you. The emergence of these thoughts is one of the most important aspects of Medical Meditation. The thoughts represent a release of energy from the subconscious mind, to the conscious mind. Each time it happens, accept it. I've been meditating for twenty-five years, and this happens every day.

If you accept this, meditation will take you to what I call the Fourth State. The Fourth State is elevated above the other three common states of mind: the awake state, the sleep state, and the dream state. The Fourth State is the transcendent state. It creates the sacred space in which all healing occurs.

Medical Meditation as Sadhana

As you can see, the process of meditation is quite simple. It becomes rather more difficult when you add the elements of kundalini yoga, and do Medical Meditations. However, Medical Meditations are more rewarding and involving.

Medical Meditations, all of which include elements of kundalini yoga, are presented in this book in a self-explanatory format. To perform them, you will simply have to read about the meditations, and follow the instructions and the drawings that accompany them.

For many people, one of the greatest challenges of Medical Meditation is to integrate meditation wholly into the fabric of their lives. Part of doing this is participating in a regular morning program of yoga and meditation. I call this morning program Wake Up to Wellness. The ancient masters called it *sadhana* (pronounced "SOD-nuh").

Some patients have told me they could never wake up early in the morning and do meditative yoga. But they tried it—and it paid off. So they stuck with it. It was purely a matter of following their own self-interest. Yogi Bhajan finds sadhana so personally rewarding that he calls it a totally selfish act. He says that it gives him personal strength, intuition, sharpness, dignity, and grace.

A student once asked him, "Sir, you're a master, why do you still do sadhana?"

He replied, "Because I want to stay a master."

Deepak Chopra, M.D., begins his practice of sadhana almost every day at 4:00 A.M. I asked him once if he found it difficult, and he said, "I enjoy it! Without it, I certainly wouldn't be as healthy, happy, or successful as I am."

Personally, I couldn't imagine life without my daily practice of sadhana. To me, it is the key to higher living, the kind of living I do when I am in the flow, and in touch with my highest self. It is much more than just a physical and mental tune-up. It is so utterly fulfilling that it can be most accurately described as a spiritual experience.

SADHANA

For some people, the hardest part of sadhana is getting up early in the morning. This is not absolutely essential, but it is manifestly helpful. Here is what a great sixteenth-century master, Guru Amardas, said about rising early for sadhana: "The dawn of the day is the ambrosial hour, when nature is flowing its peerless fragrance in full splendor, and the mind and soul of man are crystal clear, because the dust of the day's entanglements has not affected them yet. When the seeker prays from his heart in the ambrosial hours, he is blessed with the Lord's grace."

It is my theory that the ambrosia that the ancient masters spoke of was a metaphorical reference to the endocrine secretions the body produces at this time of day. These secretions begin with the actions of the hypothalamus and the pituitary gland, which then orchestrate the symphony of the rest of the endocrine system. When these secretions are produced in a state of calmness, with heightened awareness, they tend to be optimally balanced. This powerfully inhibits the common mood disorders of depression and anxiety.

When I first started doing sadhana, in 1981, I would get up at 5:00 A.M., take a shower, and practice for thirty minutes to an hour. Sometimes I would finish by taking a hot tub, and getting a bite to eat. I could have gotten up later, but I discovered that sadhana gave me much more energy than extra sleep.

At the very beginning of my practice, I did only about twenty minutes of kundalini yoga and eleven minutes of meditation. Since then, I've found that the more I do, the better I feel, so I am now more disciplined. Presently my sadhana is about one and a half to two hours long. When you first begin, you may want to do only a short sadhana, as I initially did. The key is to begin now, and to do at least something every day. Don't pressure yourself. Don't label yourself good if you do a lot and bad if you don't. Those labels are artificial and counterproductive. Your goal should be joy—not logging as many hours as possible.

Note, for example, how quickly positive effects occur during Medical Meditation:

3 MINUTES: Increased blood circulation begins, distributing enhanced neuroendocrine secretions throughout the body.

7 MINUTES: Brain patterns begin to shift from the static of beta waves, to calmer alpha waves, and ultimately to deep-relaxation delta waves. Simultaneously, the magnetic force surrounding the body increases in strength.

11 MINUTES: The sympathetic and parasympathetic nervous systems begin to accommodate increased energy.

22 MINUTES: Anxiety-producing thoughts in the subconscious begin to clear.

31 MINUTES: Endocrinological balance is achieved, as is balance of the chakras of the ethereal body. This balance persists throughout the day, and is reflected by changes in mood and behavior.

Following is a sample sadhana routine, one I use myself and recommend to patients.

THE STRUCTURE OF SADHANA

- Your sadhana actually starts the night before. Eat lightly, and as early as you comfortably can. A heavy, late meal is a sadhana-buster. It's harder to focus during meditation while you're still digesting food.
- Go to bed at a reasonable hour, such as 10:00 P.M. As you're drifting into sleep, pray to your highest self for help in waking up in the ambrosial hours.
- Move your bowels either the night before, or upon arising. This increases your flexibility and enhances mental focus.
- Rise before dawn in the *amrit vela,* "time of nectar," traditionally between 4:00 A.M. and 7:00 A.M. Perhaps a good time for beginners is around 5:00 A.M. or 6:00 A.M. Early rising is preferable, but be sure to take time for your sadhana whenever you arise. If you just don't have time in the morning, you can do it in the evening, but you will experience much less of a carry-over effect into your normal workday.

- Lightly massage your body with almond oil and take a shower. Spiritual tradition recommends a cold shower, which shifts blood flow from your skin to your inner organs, and stimulates the nervous system. Many people start with warm water, and gradually cool it. Wrap yourself in a comfortable robe or towel.
- Wear comfortable, stretchy clothing.
- If you're hungry, eat something light, such as a piece of fruit, or part of a protein bar.
- Eliminate all possible distractions, go to a quiet place, and sit on a surface that's comfortable, but not too soft.
- Tune in by chanting the Adi Mantra: "Ong Namo Guru Dev Namo" ("I bow before my highest self"). As you chant this, sit cross-legged, with your spine straight. Press your palms together, with your fingers pointed up. Inhale deeply, and focus your attention on your third-eye point. As you exhale, chant the mantra in one breath. If you can't do it in one breath, take a short breath after *Ong Namo*. The sound *Dev* is chanted at a slightly higher tone than the other sounds. As you chant, vibrate your cranium enough to create mild pressure at the third-eye point. Chant this mantra at least three times. For the best effect, do it to the simple tune:

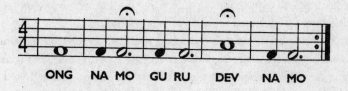

ONG   NA MO   GU RU   DEV   NA MO

- Do 5–10 minutes of personal prayer, affirmations, and goal setting. Focus especially on what you hope to achieve during this session of sadhana, and this day.
- Say a short formal prayer that is true to your religion or philosophy.
- Do 10–30 minutes of stretching and breath work to invigorate your body and to rid yourself of physical distractions. You may want to use the physical Medical Meditation found at the end of this chapter to start your day.
- Relax for 2–5 minutes by lying down and paying attention to your breath.
- Do the morning call found on page 148, or your Medical

Meditations. You may do only one meditation, if appropriate, or you may do more than one.

- Relax again, and try to connect your relaxed, empowered mood to the one that you will carry into your day. One way to do this is to sing a simple, spiritual song, such as "May the Longtime Sun Shine upon You," which is found at the end of this chapter.

By the time you finish this, the morning will be in its full glory, all will be right with your world, and you will be at peace.

SADHANA AS ITS OWN REWARD

For people like my patient Jane, the effort of sadhana is its own reward. Jane, as you'll recall, didn't have a major, acute pathology, but had a general deficiency syndrome characterized by low energy, malaise, muscle aches, and insomnia. Her essential malady, I thought, was not just biochemical, or even psychological. It went deeper than that. Her problems weren't just in her body and mind, but in her spirit, too. Over the course of her life, she'd faced too many challenges that she just couldn't handle. Each one took something out of her. Her physical, emotional, and spiritual decline had been gradual, as it usually is for the millions of people who suffer from this syndrome and are labeled neurotic or hypochondriacal. One day she'd simply woken up feeling half-dead and couldn't remember ever feeling different.

By the time she'd sunk to that level, she had a profound inability to internalize, circulate, and release life energy, or prana. For her, trying to get enough prana was like an emphysema patient trying to get enough oxygen.

But all that changed when she began to do Medical Meditation. I urged her to perform a rigorous program of sadhana, and at first she rebelled against the idea. She thought that requiring more energy from her poor depleted body was foolish, since it didn't have enough to begin with. But that's the beauty of energy—the more you put out, the more you get back! This is particularly true when you do activities like sadhana that are specifically designed to increase energy.

When Jane began to feel the first stirrings of her old energy—that restless joy that begs for activity—she was shocked. She felt, she said, as if she were creating something out of nothing.

But Jane wasn't a nothing. She was just empty. As long as individuals have life, though, no matter how empty they are, they can still find their way to power and grace. The secret is simply to reach inside yourself, and grasp the teeming, seething energy that exists inside you. It is there, waiting for you.

By practicing sadhana, with its daily Medical Meditations, Jane had allowed this cosmic energy to circulate in her. With it, she was reborn—spiritually, physically, and psychologically. Of course, there was a physical manifestation of this rebirth: her adrenal glands became more active, her production of the neurotransmitters norepinephrine and dopamine increased, and her thyroid function, according to a panel of blood tests, improved notably. However, to ascribe her healing to these physical changes would be medically inaccurate. Jane had healed—and then she had changed.

Now, perhaps, it is your time to heal—and then to change. The healing force is within you, and surrounds you. It is in the air. You can breathe it.

Following are several basic kriyas that I have found to be invaluable in my own morning sadhana. These may be combined with other yoga exercises and meditations, or used on their own.

Sadhana Medical Meditations

MEDICAL MEDITATIONS TO START THE DAY

Tune in and center yourself by chanting "Ong Namo, Guru Dev Namo" 3 times (Tune on page 143).

1. Posture: Lying on your back, stretch your arms at your sides with the fingers straight. Raise your feet, head, and hands off the floor, and hold the position for the length of the exercise.

Focus: Your eyes should look at your big toes.

Breath: Do Breath of Fire while holding the position.

Mantra: This Medical Meditation is done without a mantra.

Mudra: The hands are stretched and point toward your feet.

Time: Start with as little as 30 seconds; gradually you can build up to 3 minutes.

This exercise is called Stretch Pose. Make sure your back is flat on the floor. If your waist does not touch the floor, then place your hands beneath your hips for support. If you need to, you can take a 5-second break, but then resume the exercise. This exercise energizes the third chakra and the navel center.

2. Posture: Bend your knees and clasp your legs with your arms. Raise your head so that your nose comes between your knees.

Focus: The eyes are closed and focused at the third-eye point.

Breath: Breath of Fire.

Mantra: This Medical Meditation is done without a mantra.

Mudra: Your hands are clasped around your legs.

Time: 1–2 minutes.

This exercise stretches and relaxes the neck muscles, the area where we store all the psychic tension.

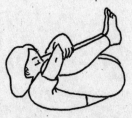

3. Posture: Same position as above, lying on your back with your knees to your chest and your nose between your knees. Roll back and forth on your spine, from neck to tailbone.

Focus: The eyes are closed and focused at the third-eye point.

Breath: Coordinate the breath with the movement.

Mantra: This Medical Meditation is done without a mantra.

Mudra: Your hands are clasped around your legs.

Time: 1 minute.

This exercise distributes pranic energy throughout your body and relaxes your back muscles.

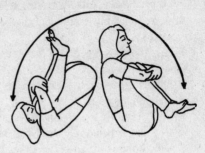

4. Posture: Sit in Easy Pose or in a chair with your spine straight.

Focus: The eyes are closed and focused at the third-eye point.

Breath: Breath of Fire.

Mantra: This Medical Meditation is done without a mantra.

Mudra: Raise your arms up to 60 degrees to the sides, fingertips in, thumbs extended out, and pointed straight up.

Time: 2 minutes.

End: Inhale deeply and hold your breath while you raise your arms up above your head until your thumbs touch. Strongly press the tips of the thumbs against each other until you cannot hold your breath in any longer. Exhale and flatten your hands, slowly arc them down, sweeping the aura with the palms, collecting any darkness, negativity, or sickness. Release it into the earth to clean and energize the aura. Feel the light around you, and meditate on that light.

This exercise is called Ego Eradicator.

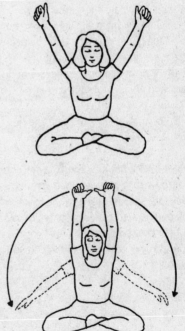

COMMENTS: This Medical Meditation may be done every morning while you are still in bed. This is an excellent set to energize you and prepare you for a great day.

MORNING CALL MEDICAL MEDITATION

This follows the Medical Meditations to Start the Day.

Posture: Sit in Easy Pose or in a chair with your spine straight. Relax your hands on your knees.

Focus: The eyes are closed and focused at the third-eye point.

Breath: Described in Mantra. All breathing is done through the nose.

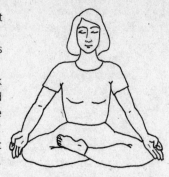

Mantra: Take a deep breath and chant "Ek Ong Kar" (the Ek being very short, the Ong and Kar being long and equal in length). Take another deep breath and chant "Sat Nam Siri" (Sat is short, Nam is very long, and Siri just escapes your tongue with the last bit of breath). Take a short breath and chant "Wa-Hey Guru" (Wahe and Gu are short, ru is long).

Meaning of mantra: This is a very powerful mantra for awakening kundalini and suspending the mind in bliss. It means there is one creative force, whose true essence is great beyond description.

Mudra: The hands are in gyan mudra, with the thumbs touching the index fingers, and are relaxed on the knees.

Time: 7–11 minutes.

End: Inhale deeply through the nose. Hold for 10 seconds. Exhale through the nose and relax.

COMMENTS: Before sunrise, when the channels of energy are most clear, if this mantra is sung in sweet harmony, you will be one with the Lord. This will open your solar plexus, charging the solar center, connecting it with cosmic energy. You will be liberated from the cycles of karma that bind you to the earth. No tongue can tell how bright the light of cosmic energy is, but when you recite this mantra daily, you will have this light within you.

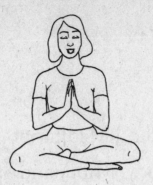

LONGTIME SUNSHINE SONG

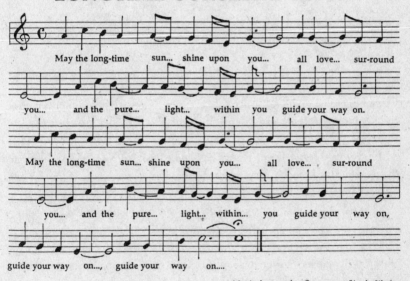

May the long-time sun... shine upon you... all love... sur-round you... and the pure... light... within you guide your way on.

May the long-time sun... shine upon you... all love... sur-round you... and the pure... light... within... you guide your way on, guide your way on..., guide your way on....

Musical score by Guruprem Singh Khalsa

CHAPTER NINE

Medical Meditation Heals Body, Mind, and Spirit

Nicole's Story

One of my most memorable patients ever was Nicole, whom I mentioned at the beginning of the book. Nicole, a gifted photographer, was just twenty-three; beautiful and charismatic, she had always faced the life ahead of her as if it were a shining dawn. Things had come easily to Nicole, and she'd had the type of magnetic, enveloping charm that had made people happy for her, instead of envious.

Then her luck had reversed, with the shocking suddenness that sometimes seems to befall only those who have it all.

One day, Nicole had been photographing a speeding train, edging ever closer to it, closer, closer, to capture an angle that made the long train seem to narrow to a spear point as it receded into the distance.

Then: cataclysm! An explosion of fury! She was rammed from behind by an irresistible force. Another train, hidden from sight, and hidden from sound by the roar of the train she was photographing, had rushed up behind her. It smashed into her, and she cartwheeled across the hard gravel.

Nicole lay facedown, immobile, still conscious, as searing waves of pain shuddered up and down her body.

When her friends found her, she was lying between the two sets of tracks, bloody and broken. One of her lungs was collapsed, her wrists were shattered, and her liver, kidneys, and spleen were pummeled and bleeding internally. Worst of all, Nicole's back was broken, and her spinal cord had been stretched like a rubber band, destroying its ability to transmit nerve impulses.

For six days, Nicole was incoherent and feverish as she struggled for life.

She finally came fully awake in a strange world of pain, fog, and paralysis. She was crushed: mentally and physically and spiritually.

When the most acute danger of death passed, Nicole was air-evacuated to a rehabilitation center in Colorado. Endless weeks of sheer torture produced little improvement. She had no feeling or movement from her chest down. When she left rehab, she was confined to a wheelchair.

She had tried to hold out hope during her rehabilitation, but it had not been well received by her doctors. She had been urged to live in the real world. But for her, this was now a world of helplessness and never-ending agony. She was desperate for something better. She longed for her old life. That life seemed real to her—not this ugly new one.

According to what she'd already said to me during our first conversation, a telephone call, she was praying I could work wonders, and bring life back to her legs. She had already consulted with two of America's most renowned healers, Deepak Chopra, M.D., and Andrew Weil, M.D., and they had awakened her to the extraordinary possibilities of the body's own self-healing. But they really hadn't been able to help. Her injuries were just too extensive. Dr. Weil had referred her to me because he hoped that I could help with her severe, intractable pain.

When I first looked into Nicole's eyes, the dark specter of death haunted them, and seemed to form a swirling vortex of fear that drew life in and never let it out. Somewhere in those two black holes was Nicole, alone and cold. I took her hand, and it chilled mine.

"Dr. Khalsa," she said from her wheelchair, looking trapped in it, "help me to walk again."

I didn't know what to say.

"Please!" she said emphatically, as if desperation itself could mint power.

Nicole had been too close to death too often—not only from the accident, but also from her many dangerous surgeries, which would number eighteen over five and a half years—and now death seemed to hold her in its sway. This fed her fear, day and night, as did the constant threat of ever more pain.

Almost as terrifying to Nicole as death and pain, though, was the prospect of a life of lost freedom. She and I began to talk quietly about the beauty of the desert, and I found she had a religious communion with nature. It was her church, and now she was virtually banned from it. No longer could she walk in solitude among the trees, rocks, and rivers that had once lit her with life.

With heartrending regret in her voice, she said, "If I could just go back to that train track, and be a little more careful, none . . ."

I cut her off gently. "Nicole," I said softly, "you can't go back. You can only go forward."

"I know. It just makes me so mad!"

"At life?"

"At me. At the engineer of the train that hit me, 'cuz he was going too fast. Yeah, and at life, too." Her jaw clenched, and her face hardened.

"When we start working together," I said, "I'll try to help you find a way to use the feelings that hurt you now, like your fear and anger. I'll show you how to make them empower your healing."

"To regenerate my nerves?" she asked hopefully. "I've heard you're doing amazing things with neurological regeneration."

"Maybe to regenerate your nerves, but not necessarily. My ultimate goal for you is to help you do your absolute best with what you have. If you can do that, you'll reach what I call your highest self, and you'll be at peace. That I can promise."

She sagged, disappointed.

I told her, as forcefully as I could without hurting her, that finding peace would be harder than walking. I told her I wanted to help her heal her whole life—not just her legs.

"My life isn't paralyzed. Just my legs," she said bitterly.

But Nicole was wrong. Her life was paralyzed. She was stuck. Stuck in the past. Stuck in her fear. Stuck in her anger. Stuck in regret.

This mental and spiritual paralysis was as devastating to her as the deadened nerves in her spine. If I could set her heart free, and breathe life back into her spirit, maybe, just maybe, a miracle might happen.

If not, nothing would happen. I have treated too many patients for too long to think that someone who is trapped in a negative mental and spiritual state can achieve a physical miracle. That may be how miracles happen in movies, but it's not how they happen in medicine.

In medicine, mind, body, and spirit are one, and miraculous healing only occurs when this sacred triad is united.

To help Nicole begin to heal, I taught her how to approach the Kirtan Kriya, a particularly powerful Medical Meditation. It is performed as follows:

Nicole's Meditation

MEDICAL MEDITATION FOR HEALING MIND, BODY AND SPIRIT

Tune in and center yourself chanting "Ong Namo, Guru Dev Namo" 3 times. (Tune on page 143).

Posture: Sit in Easy Pose or in a chair with your spine straight. Relax your hands on your knees.

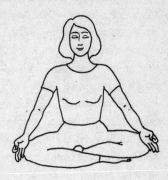

Focus: This is called the L-form meditation. With each syllable you chant, visualize that energy is flowing in through the top of your head and out your third-eye point. The eyes are closed.

Breath: The breath will come automatically as you chant.

Mantra: Sa, Ta, Na, Ma.

Meaning of mantra: This mantra represents the cycle of creation. *Sa* means infinity; *Ta* means life; *Na* means death; *Ma* means rebirth.

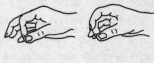

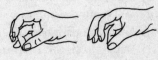

Mudra: On Sa touch the index finger to your thumb; on Ta touch the middle finger to your thumb; on Na touch the ring finger to your thumb; on Ma touch the little finger to your thumb. Apply a two-pound pressure every time you touch the fingers. Continue moving the fingers throughout the exercise, even during the silent part.

Chant in a normal voice for 2 minutes, then whisper for 2 minutes, then go deep within yourself for 3 minutes (and still continue to repeat the mantra). Come back to the whisper for 2 minutes, and finally to the normal voice for 2 minutes.

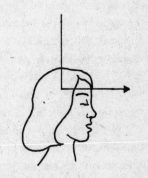

Time: 11 minutes total.

End: Inhale completely, then exhale all the air. Stretch your hands up as far as possible and spread them wide. Stretch your spine up and take several deep breaths.

COMMENTS: Practicing this Medical Meditation brings a total mental balance to the individual's mind. Other positive effects are increased concentration, enhanced creativity, and greater intuition.

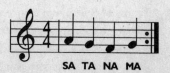

SA TA NA MA

I began to tell Nicole how Medical Meditation impacted the physical body and the ethereal body (including the chakras). I told her that there was a literal meaning to these primal sounds—Sa, Ta, Na, Ma, "birth, life, death, and rebirth." Furthermore, when these sounds were combined, they formed the phrase "Sat Nam ("my true identity," or "highest self"). These concepts were the mental focus of this Medical Meditation. Concentrating on these concepts would free her mind, at least temporarily, from fear and anger. It would also help pattern her thinking into a positive outlook, much as cognitive therapy would. Being free from fear and anger, and feeling more positive, would have a notable effect upon her nervous system. She would become less dominated by the stimulating, fight-or-flight sympathetic branch of her central nervous system, and more influenced by the healing, rest-and-repair parasympathetic branch.

Her positive and recuperative mental state, however, would be just the beginning of her healing. The other elements of her Medical Meditation (movement, breath, finger position, and sound vibration) would powerfully reinforce the effects achieved by mental conditioning.

For example, her breathing technique would enhance blood circulation, as well as circulation of ethereal energy to her brain, which is located in the seventh chakra. It would especially send ethereal energy to a part of her brain that governed the hypothalamic-pituitary-adrenocortical axis, or HPA axis, which governs the endocrine system.

The HPA axis would also be strongly influenced by the vibrational effects of her mantra. The sounds Sa Ta Na Ma would create vibrations in the upper palate of her mouth that would transfer directly to her nearby midbrain, where the HPA axis is located. Although this naturalistic ultrasound approach may sound futuristic, advanced imaging techniques, such as MRI scans, have revealed that certain sound vibrations, when repeated for several minutes, have the capacity to change the endocrine secretions controlled by the HPA axis.

The combination of all of the elements of Nicole's Medical Meditation would exert a profound physical effect. It would change her entire profile of endocrine secretions, neurotransmitter secretions, and hormonal secretions. She would phase out of her anxious, adrenergic psychophysical condition, and drift into a calm, cholinergic healing condition.

This would, among other things, halt her overproduction of the adrenal hormone cortisol, which is often extremely elevated in people with chronic pain. It would also increase her output of the salubrious neurotransmitter serotonin, which is generally in short supply among people who have endured as much stress as Nicole had. This would in all probability markedly reduce her fear, her free-floating anxiety, and her anger.

The Kirtan Kriya, along with other meditations, would also bring increased blood flow and increased flow of ethereal energy not only to her spinal cord but also to her damaged internal organs. The meditations, including the exercises, would impact several of her chakras, and increase her spinal flexibility, her muscle tone, her breathing capacity, and her coordination. If all of these effects occurred robustly, I felt there was a chance that she might regain some of her lost neurological capabilities. Fortunately, her spinal cord had not been completely severed, so it had somewhat more of a chance of regenerating than do the cords of many people who have suffered paralyzing injuries.

All of the physical and psychological improvements would hopefully buoy Nicole's flagging spirits. That would be pivotally important, because in a situation as dire as this, the spirit is often the single most potent healing force. The spirit affects the emotions, the emotions affect the neurochemistry, and the neurochemistry affects the physical system.

Over the next several weeks, Medical Meditation seemed to nurture Nicole's body, mind, and spirit. As I'd hoped, she threw herself into it wholeheartedly. She was tough. She began to gain strength, physically, mentally, and spiritually.

I became optimistic that she had passed the worst of her crises. But sometimes I'm too optimistic.

CRISIS

I hate it when the phone rings in the middle of the night. Good news can always wait until morning. Bad news arrives on its own schedule.

"I can't sit up!" It was Nicole. Her voice was tight, strangled with anguish.

"Why not?"

"Every time I try to sit up, it feels like someone's hitting my head with an ax."

"Is it okay when you lie back down?"

"Yeah, it goes away quickly."

"It sounds like it might be a spinal headache. If it is, your spinal canal is leaking cerebrospinal fluid. I'll call the hospital. Try not to worry. We'll get it fixed."

It turned out that Nicole did have a leak in her spinal canal. She required an immediate procedure to plug it. Her own blood was injected into the space surrounding her spinal canal, and as it clotted around the lesion, it plugged the leak. But an even more serious problem was discovered. A pocket of spinal fluid had collected around her spinal cord and formed a cyst. It would require an eight-to-ten-hour surgery to remove both the cyst and a substantial amount of scar tissue.

Her neurosurgeon, though, was astonished that the cyst had not caused significantly more damage, by blocking the flow of cerebrospinal fluid in her spinal cord. According to the tenets of Western medicine, there was no way to explain this—it had been a miracle.

But there was, of course, an explanation. Nicole had been doing Medical Meditations that were specifically designed to increase the flow of cerebrospinal fluid in her spinal cord. These meditations, which included extensive spinal flexion kundalini yoga exercises, had exerted a powerful normalizing force against the blockage caused by the cyst.

Before, during, and after her operation, Nicole listened to a meditation tape I prepared for her. The surgery was successful, but it was terribly hard on Nicole.

The spinal column, including the cord, is perhaps the most delicate, sensitive structure in the body, and it's just not designed to accommodate the extensive cutting, twisting, and chiseling that poor Nicole had to endure. As she lay recovering from the operation, she was hurting, exhausted, and grim. She'd been through so much, with so much more to come.

She had made a great deal of progress since I'd met her. She could sit upright with no help now, her sense of balance was far better, she had much more upper body strength and coordination, she could breathe more easily, and she had increased endurance. There was no pain that Nicole would not face, nor any part of her psyche she would not explore. She had a warrior's heart and a pilgrim's soul.

But still, there was so much sadness in her. Part of her was gone, and it wasn't just her legs—it was her very selfhood. I didn't know if it would ever come back.

As she lay in bed, with sweat from pain glistening on her face, she pushed a button to summon a nurse. Her pain medication was late, and it seemed as if her nurse was purposefully withholding it, due to an unfounded fear of Nicole becoming addicted. I went to get the nurse. She grudgingly administered the medication. There was a great deal of tension in the room, and Nicole glared at the nurse's back as she left.

Nicole looked very alone. Some of her friends had been steadfast, but others had drifted away.

Nicole sighed from deep inside. She looked down at her body, limp but still in pain. "Look what I did to myself," she said. Her voice was flat, and that made it sound all the sadder.

PROGRESS

"I need help!" Nicole said. "I have a problem." She'd made an unannounced visit to my office. But she didn't look as if she had a problem. Her blue eyes were bright, and her face looked pink and healthy.

"What kind of problem?" I asked.

"It's sore down here," she said, touching the base of her spine, barely repressing a grin.

"Sore! You can feel it?"

She nodded her head vigorously, shaking her blond curls, and the grin came all the way out. It lit the room, and made me feel warm in my chest.

"Let me check it," I said.

"Would it be easier to check," she asked, grasping the side of my desk, and pulling herself upright, "if I stood up?"

I was astonished. "How'd you do that?"

"These help." She pulled up a pant leg to reveal a heavy brace that her physical therapist had fashioned.

Now it was my turn to grin, and once I started, I couldn't stop. "Nicole! You just keep amazing me!"

Her progress really had been remarkable.

The same day I saw her, Nicole began to make arrangements for surgery to relieve the new pain in her lower back. The pain was being caused by a rod that had been inserted along her spine to help stabilize it. At first the rod had worked well because she had no feeling in that part of her body. But when feeling had begun to return, primarily as a result of her strenuous work with Medical Meditation, with it had come pain.

For the first time, though, Nicole's pain heralded healing.

* * *

Nothing lasts forever. Certainly not happiness. But happiness and sorrow, like pleasure and pain, are two sides of the same coin, and having one without the other is as impossible as having a coin with only one side.

Happiness and sorrow are the polarities that swirl the ethereal energies of the heart chakra. Both are sacred.

So when Nicole called, and told me how badly her surgery had gone, I didn't try to deny reality and hang on to my happiness.

It would be back—in time.

Lying in a hospital bed, Nicole was in so much pain that she was panting and tossing. It was as if she were being beaten by invisible fists. I took her hand, and it seemed to quiet her for a moment. She opened her eyes. Focused.

"I thought nothing could be worse than my accident," she said unevenly, with broken breaths.

Her face was sunburn-red. Her fever had spiked at 103 degrees, and was going down too slowly.

She had been through several operations in a very short period of time. The one that had been most troublesome was a spine-straightening surgery, to decrease the scoliosis she'd begun to suffer. As her muscles had grown stronger, they had pulled her spine out of alignment to a dangerous degree. Unfortunately, though, during the operation, she had become infected by bacteria that had entered her bones.

The infection was painful, and so was her recovery from the various invasive procedures. Screws that had been placed in her spine had come loose, and that hurt, too.

"I try to stay with my breathing, to quiet my mind and hold down the pain," she said, pausing intermittently. "But it's so unbearable. I can't get a breath."

A nurse with a face as immobile as wood came in and took Nicole's blood pressure and pulse—far too officiously, as far as I was concerned. When she left, Nicole said, "This place needs a spiritual housecleaning."

I laughed, and felt a surge of admiration for Nicole. Here she was, tortured and sick, but somehow able to make light of her situation.

"Nicole," I said, with complete conviction, "you're going to get through this, and after you do, you're going to do whatever you want to do."

"Walk?"

"Walk." My answer wasn't an assurance. It was a prayer. She knew me well enough to know that.

"Thanks."

Her thanks was very simple, but so heartfelt that I felt blessed by it.

I stayed with her for some time.

TRIUMPH

"Nicole is here," my secretary announced.

I looked toward the open doorway of my office, and instinctively looked down to the level of Nicole's wheelchair to meet her eyes.

But then from outside the doorway I heard a soft, rhythmical rap against the floor—someone walking slowly—and caught my breath. It was Nicole. She stood in the doorway, her hands gripping forearm-crutches, smiling back at me.

Sometimes, in the midst of deep meditation, time falls off the face of the earth, and a moment becomes eternal. Those moments, I think, may be the doorways to the eternity that almost all religions speak of.

It's not the mere freezing of time that makes these moments sacred. Time can be halted by terror, too, and even sleep. It's the unutterable peace that makes sacred these moments—the soundless sound you hear—the connectedness to a universe not described by physics.

That is the magic of these moments.

If only there were a way to walk through that door . . . and stay . . .

But that is not the nature of life.

And so, too, there came an end to the moment I first saw Nicole walk. But that moment is with me always, even now, never-ending.

Technically, Nicole was bracewalking or ambulating, not walking. But I don't care what it's called, and neither does Nicole. She was back on her feet, literally and figuratively, and that was what she needed to feel whole and healthy.

Nicole is now enrolled at the Miami Project to Cure Paralysis in Florida, where she continues to heal. She strives to walk without braces in water, sails, and is engaged to a wonderful young man. Her pain is transient and manageable.

Nicole had once been trapped in a world that held no hope—only pain, dependence, and the threat of death. Out of this, with only her spirit and the guidance of the ancient masters, she created for herself a new world.

Wahe Guru. Out of the darkness into the light.

PART THREE

Healing with the

Chakra System

CHAPTER TEN

The Chakras and
Their Dysfunctions

Now we move on. To you—and your healing. No matter your malady, it's never too late to heal. Listen to the words of a great poet, and a meditator—Alfred, Lord Tennyson—who found a new world inside himself.

> *The lights begin to twinkle from the rocks.*
> *The long day wanes, the slow moon climbs,*
> *The deep moans round with many voices.*
> *Come, my friends,*
> *'Tis not too late to seek a newer world.*

—TENNYSON

The essential mechanism of action of Medical Meditation is to nurture the ethereal energy system, which transfers this nurturance to the physical body. This transfer takes place primarily via the eight chakras.

The eight chakras consist of the seven whirling vortexes of ethereal energy that are vertically aligned along the spine and head, plus the aura of ethereal energy that surrounds the entire body. The eight chakras are active at all times, even when we are not aware of them. The chakras not only hold ethereal energy, but also transfer it to other chakras. In addition, they transmit ethereal energy to the physical body, primarily by bringing energy to nerves and endocrine glands. Each chakra is located in the exact same area as a major nerve plexus, and an important endocrine gland.

Doctors who are skeptical of the existence of chakras ascribe the apparent power that resides in these specific areas of the body solely to the nerve plexuses and endocrine glands. Of course, I consider this skepticism to be ill-informed. Nonetheless, these nerve plexuses and endocrine glands are vitally important, because they enable ethereal energy to be transmitted to the physical plane.

The beauty and elegance of the chakra system is that it is not strictly physical, nor is it completely metaphysical. Instead, it is an absolutely unique confluence of both material and nonmaterial energy. As such, it exists equally in the realms of body, mind, and spirit.

Therefore, each chakra has not only specific physical characteristics but also specific psychological and spiritual characteristics. Within each chakra, all of these characteristics, whether physical or metaphysical, resonate with similarities. For example, the first chakra, located near the rectum, is closely associated, on the physical level, with elimination of waste products. On the psychological level, it is closely associated with the elimination of negative thinking. On the spiritual level, it is associated with eliminating the illusion of isolation. Each of these characteristics, of course, influences the others, due to the unity of body, mind, and spirit. In fact, the chakras make possible the complete unity of body, mind, and spirit.

Medical Meditations further knit the unity of body, mind, and spirit by amplifying the energy that resides in the chakras. No illness exists on just the physical, or just the psychological, or just the spiritual level. For illness to exist, it must overpower the positive forces of all three levels. And the positive forces of all three levels must be restored to again overpower illness.

One important way that the chakras unite body, mind, and spirit is by transmitting ethereal energy from the lower chakras to the higher chakras. They transmit this energy, or prana, through the system of nadis, the nonphysical energy conduits that are somewhat like acupuncture meridians. There are three main nadis: one is the *ida,* which correlates to the left nostril, and runs down the left side of the spine, carrying a cooling, feminine, relaxing, yin type of energy. The second is the *pingala,* which correlates to the right nostril, and runs down the right side of the spine, carrying a warming, masculine, excitatory, yang type of energy. After these two types of energy are drawn into the body, primarily through breath, they are carried by the ida and the pingala to the base of the spine, where the first chakra resides. This energy is then swirled in the vortex of the first chakra by the polarities that exist there. For example, in the first chakra, the polarities include the desire for individuality versus the desire for companionship. When this prana is swirled by polarity, it increases in strength and becomes kundalini energy: the healing energy. This kundalini is then carried back up the spine by the central nadi, the *shushmana,* the energy channel that runs up the center of the spine. The kundalini energy that rises through the shushmana can be carried to any one of the other seven chakras. It can also activate physical energy in the spinal cord, through vibrational resonance.

It's vitally important that kundalini be stimulated to rise. If it is allowed to remain in the lowest chakra, or first chakra, this chakra can dominate a person's entire life. In fact, it's quite common for people to have too much energy in their lower chakras—particularly in the first, second, and third chakras. When this occurs, people become far too fixated on the characteristics associated with those chakras. The lower chakras are primarily involved with the base elements of material life, such as survival, power, financial security, and procreation. In contrast, the four higher chakras, and the aura (or eighth chakra), are far more involved with the higher, more advanced elements of life, such as compassion, intuition, intellect, selfless service, and spirituality.

Because of the stark contrasts between the lower and higher chakras, the chakra system is often described as consisting of the lower triangle (the first, second, and third chakras), and the upper triangle (the fourth, fifth, sixth, seventh, and eighth chakras).

The lower triangle, plus the fourth and fifth chakras, have less lofty associations than the very highest chakras—the sixth, seventh, and eighth chakras, which are intricately linked to the mind and spirit. Therefore, each of the first five chakras is connected with an emotional obstacle to enlightenment. These obstacles, or negative emotions, are heightened by unbalanced energy within the chakra. The obstacles were named *tattwas* by the ancient masters. The tattwa of the first chakra is attachment. The tattwa of the second chakra is lust. The third: greed. The fourth: pride. The fifth: anger.

Even though these tattwas can be negative, they are fundamental to the human condition, and can be of valuable service. The negativity of the five tattwas mixes with the positive elements in the five lower chakras, creating a swirl of polarities that increases the chakras' energies, just as colliding warm air and cool air create the energetic vortex of an updraft.

The energy that is created by this mixture of polarities can even be used to overcome the tattwas' innate negativity. The human spirit can use the chakra's augmented energy, for example, to transform ordinary anger into righteous indignation. Similarly, sexual lust can be transformed into a healthy lust for life.

When energy moves freely among the chakras, it stimulates the mental, physical, and spiritual health of the entire organism. However, when energy becomes stuck, the organism loses its balance, or homeostasis. This depresses physical and mental energy, impairs immunity, and contributes to aging.

Energy is most likely to get stuck in the lower chakras, because it's easy to become bogged down in the daily struggle for survival and security. Unfortunately, though, happiness is not to be found in the lower chakras. When the lower chakras control us, we are separated from our higher selves, and suffer from the illusions that haunt the material world. Trapped in the lower chakras, we believe that life is finite, that survival is a constant struggle, and that we are alone.

As Shakti Parwha Kaur Khalsa noted in her book *Kundalini: The Flow of Power*, the three most important elements of kundalini energy are location, location, and location. If your kundalini energy is located in your higher chakras, you will thrive. If it's stagnating in your lower chakras, your life, like the lives of so many others, will be dross and difficult. It will be myopically focused upon the loss of the past, the fear of the future, and the drudgery of making a living.

This certainly doesn't mean, though, that the lower chakras are of no value. As Dr. Gurucharan Singh Khalsa has written, "No chakra stands alone. They are all part of a larger cycle of evolution and devolution, manifestation and sublimation. The function of elimination and reduction is balanced by the upper areas, which accumulate, create, and differentiate."

When kundalini energy does rise from the lower chakras to the higher chakras, it is an extraordinary experience. I have experienced this many, many times, but each time it happens, there is a sense of newness and wonder to it. One of the best, and most commonly used descriptions of this experience is that it is like being born once again.

Scientific Evidence of the Chakras

Even though the chakras are nonphysical, their existence has nonetheless been identified by a number of researchers. In one of the most interesting experiments, Dr. Hiroshi Motoyama of Japan placed subjects in a lead-lined booth that was shielded from electromagnetic energy, and then measured human bioelectric energy in the chakra areas of his subjects. Some of the subjects were advanced meditators, and some were not. All of the subjects exhibited increased bioelectric energy in the area of their chakras. Furthermore, when the advanced meditators focused their energies upon certain chakras, those chakras emanated significantly more bioelectric energy. This led Dr. Motoyama to conclude that the meditators had the ability to consciously activate their own chakras. Dr. Motoyama replicated this experiment several times, and so did another independent researcher.

In another revealing experiment, conducted by Dr. Valerie Hunt at UCLA, EMG electrodes, connected to telemetry equipment, were used to detect energy in chakras. Dr. Hunt noted distinct high-frequency oscillations coming from the chakra areas. The oscillations occurred at up to 1,600 cycles per second, compared to the body's usual oscillations of approximately 200 cycles per second.

In another fascinating phase of the experiment, Dr. Hunt enlisted the services of one of America's most prominent spiritual healers, Rosalyn Bruyere. Among Bruyere's gifts is the ability to actually see a person's aura, or eighth chakra. Although this ability may sound exotic, it's a talent that many people have been able to learn (though few have mastered it as well as Bruyere). In the experiment, Bruyere visually noted changes in the color and intensity of the subjects' auras, while Dr. Hunt monitored the subjects electronically. Dr. Hunt found that the changes noticed by Bruyere corresponded exactly to changes in oscillation frequency picked up by the technological equipment.

The Chakras and Their Dysfunctions

To get a sense of the big picture of the chakra system, study the following chart. For simplicity's sake, the chart is compartmentalized. In the day-to-day functioning of the chakras, though, these neat compartments become rather more blurred, as adjacent chakras affect one another, and as energy flows from chakra to chakra.

THE CHAKRAS

NUMBER OF CHAKRA	SANSKRIT NAME	LOCATION OF CHAKRA	ASSOCIATED ELEMENT	ASSOCIATED NERVOUS SYSTEM STRUCTURE	ASSOCIATED ENDOCRINE STRUCTURE
First chakra	*Muladhara* ("root")	Base of spine	Earth	Coccygeal plexus	Gonads
Second chakra	*Svadhisthana*	Behind lower abdomen	Water	Sacral plexus	Leydig cells
Third chakra	*Manipura*	Behind the navel	Fire	Solar plexus	Adrenal gland
Fourth chakra	*Anahata*	Behind the heart	Air	Cardiac plexus	Thymus
Fifth chakra	*Visuddhu*	Throat	Ether	Laryngeal plexus	Thyroid
Sixth chakra	*Ajna* ("sun")	Center of forehead or third-eye point		Brain	Pituitary gland
Seventh chakra	*Sahasrara* ("crown")	Top of head		Brain	Pineal gland
Eighth chakra		Aura		Bioelectric field	

THE CHAKRAS (CONTINUED)

NUMBER OF CHAKRA	ASSOCIATED ORGANS OR PHYSICAL STRUCTURES	ASSOCIATED TATTWA	ASSOCIATED PSYCHOLOGICAL AND SPIRITUAL CHARACTERISTICS	ASSOCIATED PATHOLOGIES
First chakra	Colon; rectum; spine; legs	Attachment	Ego; survival; isolation; elimination; companionship	Colorectal pathology, including cancer; constipation
Second chakra	Sex organs; bladder; pelvis	Lust	Creativity; guilt; anxiety about money	Sciatica; pelvic, urinary, and gynecological problems; sexual dysfunction
Third chakra	Stomach; liver; kidneys	Greed	Power; strength; transformation; self-esteem	Ulcers; stomach, intestinal, and liver problems; adrenal problems
Fourth chakra	Heart; lungs; thymus	Pride	Love; grief; forgiveness; trust; optimism	Heart problems; lung problems; breast cancer; impaired immunity
Fifth chakra	Throat; thyroid; mouth; hypothalamus	Anger	Truthfulness; decisiveness; willpower	Throat problems, including laryngitis, and laryngeal and esophageal cancer; low energy; TMJ pain
Sixth chakra	Brain; eyes		Intuition; intellectuality; confidence	Brain problems, including Alzheimer's, brain cancer, and impaired thinking; psychological disturbances
Seventh chakra	Cerebral cortex; pineal gland		Intuition; cognition; spirtuality	Psychological and cognitive problems; chronic fatigue; hypersensitivity
Eighth chakra	Skin		Spiritual unity with universe; protective "force field"	Vulnerability to pathogens; physical and mental weakness

THE CHAKRAS (CONTINUED)

NUMBER OF CHAKRA	ASSOCIATED COLOR	ASSOCIATED MUDRA OR FINGER	UNIVERSAL OR PLANETARY ASSOCIATION
First chakra	Red		Saturn
Second chakra	Orange	Index finger	Jupiter
Third chakra	Yellow	Middle finger	Mars
Fourth chakra	Green	Ring finger	Venus
Fifth chakra	Blue		Mercury
Sixth chakra	Indigo		Sun
Seventh chakra	Violet		
Eighth chakra	White		

AILMENT/CHAKRA/MEDICAL MEDITATION CHART

(SAMPLES ARE GIVEN IN THIS CHART—PLEASE REFER TO TEXT FOR ALL THE MEDICAL MEDITATIONS)

AILMENT	CHAKRA	MEDICAL MEDITATION / PAGE	COMMENT
Addictions	3rd, 7th, 8th	For habituation or addiction 269 For healing 183	Make sure thumbs are in temple niche. Works quickly. Very empowering. Brings energy up.
Age-associated memory impairment	6th, 7th, 8th	To increase cognitive function 250, 258	More effective than any drug or vitamin.
Allergies	4th	For immune system 219 For thymus gland 222	Brings the immune system into balance.
Alzheimer's disease	6th, 7th, 8th	To increase cognitive function 250, 258	There is hope. Don't rely on drug therapy alone.
Anger	1st, 4th	To release the past 182, 223	Defrost frozen anger and heal yourself.
Antiaging	5th, 6th	For 5th chakra 231 For 6th chakra 249	Sadhana. Almost all meditations are antiaging; these two are specific.
Anxiety disorder	4th, 6th	Neutral mind 217 Calm heart 218 For 6th chakra 249	Sadhana. Don't worry; don't hurry.
Cancer	4th	For immune system; thymus gland 219, 222 Healing self 272 Guru Ram Das mantra 121	Healthy am I. Happy am I. Holy am I.

AILMENT	CHAKRA	MEDICAL MEDITATION / PAGE	COMMENT
Chronic fatigue	4th; all need energy	To recharge 251 For mental fatigue 254	A good sadhana.
Chronic pain	4th, 6th; all need energy	Healing self 272 To balance and recharge 251	All healing comes from within.
Depression	6th	Sodarshan 273 Opening the higher centers 232 For depression 256	Depression is lack of spiritual connection, and anger turned in.
Diabetes	3rd	To strengthen the pancreas 204	Eliminate simple sugar and processed food.
Digestion	3rd	For digestion 202, 203	Breathwalk.
Distant healing	6th, 7th, 8th	Transferring healing energy 271 Healing others 272	Prana colored with pure intention. Projected with love.
Emphysema and other lung disorders	4th	All breathing exercises, chapter four, 72–76	The Breath of Life is your gift from God.
Epilepsy	6th	For epilepsy 253	Meditation will help your brain heal.
Fear	1st, 4th	To release fear 257	All fear is the fear of death . . . change your brain chemistry.
Fibromyalgia	4th	For immune system 219 For thymus gland 222	Always start with sadhana.
Gall-bladder disease	3rd	For 3rd chakra 201 For gall bladder problems 203	Stop eating fat. Release your anger.

AILMENT	CHAKRA	MEDICAL MEDITATION / PAGE	COMMENT
Heart disease	4th	To prevent heart attack 221 For a calm heart 218 To repair stress damage 206	It takes only a moment to open your heart and feel the love in you. A calm heart and a peaceful life is the best prescription against heart disease.
Hepatitis and chronic liver disease	3rd	Cleanse the liver 203 For 3rd chakra 201	Let the liver live. Add a diet of mung beans, rice, daikon radishes, and beets.
High blood pressure	4th; others	For high blood pressure 220	High blood pressure is directly related to how constricted you are. Meditate every day.
Insomnia		For 7th & 8th chakras 268 Basic relaxation response 139	Try a banana at bedtime.
Intuition	6th	All 6th, 7th, 8th chakras 240–74	Get in the flow and you will know.
Intuition and creativity	6th	To heal mind, body, and spirit 153	"Anyone practicing this kriya for 2½ hours a day for 1 year shall know the unknown and see the unseen." —*Yogi Bhajan*
Kidney disease	2nd	For 2nd chakra 193 For kidneys 205 For lower triangle 206	Drink pure water. Keep your energy clear.
Low self-esteem	4th	For bliss 234	Good self-esteem is a blessing. You can create it.
Menopause and/or menstrual irregularity	2nd	For menstrual irregularity 194	Also brings a stable sense of balance.

AILMENT	CHAKRA	MEDICAL MEDITATION / PAGE	COMMENT
Migraine headaches	6th	For migraine headaches 255	Raise your serotonin levels.
Mood swings	Various, 4th, 6th	Sadhana 146–149	Conquer your mind and you'll conquer the world.
Multiple sclerosis	4th, 6th, 7th	Sadhana 146–149 For 7th chakra 268	Mind-body exercise works well for MS.
Obsessive-compulsive disorder	Various	For 4th chakra 216	Calm your heart. Calm your mind. Calm your spirit.
Parathyroid disease	5th	For parathyroid imbalance 239	The glands are guardians of health.
PMS	2nd	For menstrual Irregularity and PMS 194	PMS is not a Prozac deficiency.
Prostate problems including swelling and cancer	2nd	Healing energy 183	You can prevent and treat prostate problems with Medical Meditation.
Psoriasis	4th, 8th	For immune system 219 For thymus gland 222	Deep relaxation can clear it. Mindfulness meditation scientifically proven.
Relation-ships	4th	For a calm heart 217 Resolving issues from the past 223	Doing sadhana and meditation together is the most beautiful couple therapy.
Sexual dysfunction	2nd	Sat Kriya 183 For 2nd chakra 193	Sexual dysfunction is not a Viagra deficiency.
Spiritual growth	4th, 5th, 6th, 7th, 8th	Sadhana 146–149 Open crown 270 Sodarshan 274	Please do your sadhana and pray that you live your dharma. Dharma eats up karma.

AILMENT	CHAKRA	MEDICAL MEDITATION / PAGE	COMMENT
Stress	All chakras	Sadhana 146–149 For stress relief 223	When you realize your divine nature, you see God in everything.
Stroke	6th, 7th, 8th	Heal mind, body, spirit 153 Heal self 272	Helpful as speech therapy.
Thyroid diseases	5th	For 5th chakra 231 Two meditations for opening the higher centers 232 For the thyroid 238	Knowing the truth is important. Living truth is more important still.
Ulcers	3rd	See digestion 202	Medical Meditation is a soothing balm for ulcers.

CHAPTER ELEVEN

The First Chakra

The Seat of Survival

A Case History

HEALING WITH THE FIRST CHAKRA

The patient, Phil, a twenty-eight-year-old male, came to me with intense pain in his perineum, the small, nerve-packed area of tissue between the anus and the sex organs. He had previously consulted physicians who had ruled out muscle strain, as well as prostate cancer, which ran in his family. He had consulted other practitioners of complementary medicine who unsuccessfully treated the pain with homeopathic tinctures.

Phil, a record industry executive, was diagnosed as suffering from a systemic overgrowth of *Candida albicans,* or yeast infection, with accompanying adrenal insufficiency. These conditions were largely relieved with dietary change (including a yeast-free, sugar-free diet), herbal therapy, and acupuncture. However, the perineal pain persisted, along with a nagging feeling of heaviness in the perineum.

The patient responded quite favorably, though, to a program of regular Medical Meditation. He began to do the Sat Kriya every day as part of his daily routine, or sadhana. When he did this, the perineal pain decreased notably, but still persisted in a milder form. At that point the patient was diagnosed with chronic male pelvic distress syndrome, a relatively common stress reaction that causes pain in the perineum due to spasm of the deep muscles of the pelvis, including the psoas muscle.

Phil then began to perform Medical Meditations specifically designed to bring healing energy to the first chakra. During one particularly intense session of meditation, the patient had a vivid recollection of being three years old, and suffering a severe double hernial rupture, caused by a weakening of the muscles in the pelvic region. Coincident to the patient's double hernia, he was suffering profound psychological distress, due to his parents' divorce. As Phil described it, "My entire family support structure was being yanked out from under me. My body mirrored that lack of support, and lack of foundation, by manifesting a double hernia."

When Phil made the connection between his current pain and the childhood trauma, his pain subsided dramatically. He has recently stated, "I see that pain now as the messenger that brought me to a new knowledge of self."

The pain has not returned, and Phil continues to practice Medical Meditation assiduously.

The General Characteristics of the First Chakra

The first chakra, located at the base of the spine, near the rectum, is our closest connection to the energies of the earth. It is, in a sense, our most human chakra, because it is the primary ethereal manifestation of our most primal self. As such, it is the chakra that is most distanced from our spirit.

The first chakra, characterized by the earth element, is more caught up in the realm of the senses than any other chakra. It is the first chakra to receive prana from the outside world, and is thus closely connected to the world. The prana that enters the first chakra comes, as I mentioned, via the ida and pingala nadis, which are activated by breath. The ida and pingala, as complementary opposites, bring polarized qualities of prana to the first chakra, where these qualities mix, increase in energy, and become balanced. Without this balance, the healing kundalini energy that is produced in the first chakra cannot be fully realized, and then stimulated to rise to the higher chakras. Therefore, balance, achieved primarily through breath, is vitally important to the first chakra.

When the earth element is out of balance, a person will tend to have an obsessive personality, and will often repeat behaviors from the past, which are generally destructive. If people are not grounded by the earth element, the lessons of life just don't stick, thus prompting a need for ceaseless repetition.

The first chakra, of all the chakras, is most vulnerable to missing life's lessons because it is our least reflective chakra, greatly distanced from the higher, more contemplative energy centers. As such, the first chakra is the primary repository of our unconscious urges and automatic instincts.

Reflecting the root essence of our selfhood, the first chakra is tightly bound to the survival instinct. It is, in a sense, a very pragmatic chakra, which processes every issue with an eye to the bottom line. With a strong eliminative function, the first chakra breaks every concern down to its most basic components, and then preserves the positive elements and eliminates the negative.

Dr. Gurucharan Singh Khalsa draws an analogy between the metaphysical function of the first chakra and its physical function, as the eliminator of waste products (through the rectum). When food first enters the body, he notes, we are extremely aware of its subtle qualities—its taste, texture, smell, and color. By the time this food is ready to be returned to earth, however, it has been broken down into its most basic components. It is reduced to what is most common and universal, devoid of any subtlety. This same function holds true, in the larger sense, with the metaphysical activities of the first chakra. The first chakra reduces our many varied needs and desires down to the one that is most primal: the desire to stay alive, as an individual self.

Unfortunately, energy often becomes stuck in the first chakra, due to our overriding preoccupation with survival and selfhood. When this happens, an excess of energy builds up in the first chakra. This excess of energy can cause a person to live in his or her first chakra, without bringing energy upward to the more spiritual and intellectual energy centers. This is, in a sense, a form of consciousness constipation.

When this occurs, people become far too fixated on mere biological survival, at the expense of spiritual survival. They worry too much about their health, their money, and their status. This excessive attachment to the material world keeps them from achieving the blissful condition of the neutral mind, in which they can accept any fate and still be happy. Instead they become obsessed with negative first-chakra emotions such as greed, retaliation, jealousy, and revenge. They also often begin to feel terribly isolated, imprisoned by their own exaggerated selfhood. At its worst, this feeling of isolation can devolve into paranoia.

However, when energy is flowing freely in and out of the first chakra, people are able to benefit from the best qualities that the first chakra has to offer. Among them is the elimination of negative thoughts and bad habits.

Another is the sense of security and stability that comes with having a strong sense of self. Yet another is the merging of the self with other selves, in the human drive for companionship, family, and group protection.

Physical Characteristics of the First Chakra

On the strictly physical level, energy imbalance in the first chakra can lead to problems in any of the physical structures that are associated with this chakra: the sacrum, the lower spine, the rectum, the descending colon, the anus, and the Leydig cells (which produce testosterone, and are also strongly influenced by the second chakra).

The most common of these problems are those associated with the colon, particularly the lower portion of the descending colon. Among the most feared is colorectal cancer. Colon cancer, of course, is closely related to inadequate elimination, especially of toxins. The most frequent toxic element that leads to colon cancer is animal fat. There is also evidence that environmental toxins also contribute to colon cancer.

Toxins contribute to cancer by triggering unhealthy changes in cellular DNA, the genetic coding material that enables cells to replicate themselves. As we age, the number of these replications accumulates, affording ever more opportunities for error by the DNA. Unfortunately, though, the body's DNA repair system, which is constantly on the lookout for malignant changes in cells, grows less effective as we age. Therefore, one of the prime objectives of Medical Meditation is to promote cellular, genetic integrity at the level of the DNA.

Another valuable action of Medical Meditation is to increase blood flow to specific areas, including the area of the first chakra. By promoting blood flow, and balancing energy in the first chakra, we promote health in the colon, and in the other structures associated with the first chakra.

Because colon cancer is so rampant in modern society, due largely to poor nutrition, it's wise to monitor the health of the colon regularly, particularly after age fifty. A number of tests can help discover cancerous lesions in their early stages; among them are stool tests for blood, rectal exams, sigmoidoscopies, and colonoscopies.

Less frightening than colon cancer, but still highly discomforting, are conditions such as irritable bowel syndrome, colitis, spastic colon, and Crohn's disease. These problems are not only painful in and of themselves but also compromise the assimilation of nutrients, and thereby contribute to dysfunction throughout the system.

Another serious problem associated with first chakra abnormality is chronic constipation, which is extremely common. As you know, the waste products from food are propelled through the bowel by peristaltic contractions of the colon. This muscular activity is automatic, and is thus governed by the autonomic nervous system, which is very vulnerable to stress. However, the function of the autonomic nervous system, and the organs it controls, can be greatly benefited by Medical Meditation, since it is an excellent mediator against stress. When the lower chakra is open, with energy flowing freely in and out of it, it has a powerful relaxing effect upon the nerve plexus that controls the colon. This stimulates general colonic health and helps prevent constipation.

Moreover, a lack of exercise can also lead to constipation. However, many first-chakra Medical Meditations require abdominal exercise, and significantly tone the muscles of the colon. In addition, they bring extra blood flow to the area, which also promotes the health and vitality of the colon, as well as the other first-chakra physical structures.

The first chakra (and to a larger extent, the second chakra) is also associated with the adrenal glands. The adrenals, located near the kidneys, are physically closer to the second chakra than the first chakra. However, the first chakra is intimately connected with the survival instinct, and the adrenals are the ultimate survival glands. They control the release of the fight-or-flight hormones (chiefly adrenaline and cortisol), which make survival possible during moments of crisis.

Adrenal dysfunction, in its most extreme form, results in Addison's disease, which is relatively rare. Far more common is mild adrenal insufficiency, which contributes to depression, chronic fatigue, and allergies.

If there is too much energy in the first chakra, though, it can contribute to overactivity of the adrenals. This causes agitation and anxiety. Overproduction of the adrenal hormone cortisol, as Cameron Stauth and I demonstrated in *Brain Longevity,* causes even more insidious problems. Excess cortisol accelerates the aging process, and is a major risk factor not only in Alzheimer's disease but also in the far more common condition of age-associated memory disorder.

Following are general Medical Meditations that support the first chakra, whether underactive, overactive, or balanced, and that help solve specific physical conditions associated with dysfunction of the first chakra.

Medical Meditations for the First Chakra

SPECIAL MEDITATION FOR THE FIRST CHAKRA

Tune in and center yourself by chanting "Ong Namo, Guru Dev Namo" 3 times (Tune on page 143).

Posture: Sit in Easy Pose or in a chair, making sure your spine is straight.

1. Start this Medical Meditation with your arms held out to the sides, your elbows bent and the palms of your hands facing each other at a 60-degree angle. Begin moving your hands slowly toward each other from the starting position, simultaneously squeezing the sphincter muscles of the anus, until the hands meet at the center of your body. At this time the contraction of the anus is released. Do this as a warm-up for 1–3 minutes.

2. From the starting position, bring your hands together at the center of your body (similar to clapping) in two distinct and strong moves. The first move brings your hands halfway in, as you chant Hummee Hum with the recessed tongue. Your hands stop briefly and begin to move again as you chant Brahm Hum, bringing your hands together in front of your body. When your hands move, squeeze the anus, and maintain that contraction until your hands touch. Then relax the anus, return your hands to the starting position, and begin again.

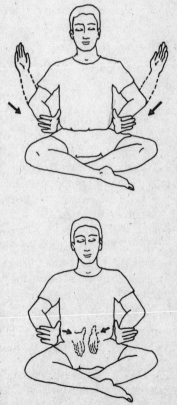

Focus: Focus your eyes at the tip of your nose.

Breath: The breath will come naturally as you chant.

Mantra: "Hummee Hum, Brahm Hum." The chanting is performed in a special way: your tongue is recessed; that is, it is relaxed and flat in the bottom of your mouth, and is not used to chant the mantra. This will produce a pressure that will be felt in the cheekbone area.

Meaning of mantra: "We are we, and we are one." On a higher spiritual level; "We are already everything we need to be."

Mudra: Your hands are open and relaxed, with the palms facing each other.

Time: Begin with 11 minutes and slowly work up to 31 minutes.

End: Inhale deeply in the starting position, hold your breath for 10 seconds, exhale, and relax.

COMMENTS: This Medical Meditation raises the kundalini energy and directs healing energy to ailments of the first chakra.

MEDICAL MEDITATION TO RELEASE
THE PAST, ESPECIALLY CHILDHOOD ANGER

Tune in and center yourself by chanting "Ong Namo, Guru Dev Namo" 3 times (Tune on page 143).

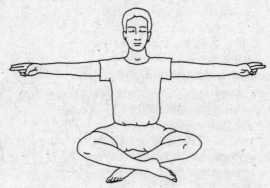

Posture: Sit in Easy Pose or in a chair, with your spine straight and chin in. Extend your arms to the sides parallel to the ground, and keep them straight.

Focus: The eyes are closed and focused at the third-eye point.

Breath: Inhale deeply by sucking air through your closed teeth and exhale through your nose. Keep your jaw relaxed.

Mantra: This Medical Meditation is done without a mantra.

Mudra: Use your thumbs to lock down the pinkie and ring fingers, and extend the index and middle fingers. The palms face forward and the fingers point out to the sides.

Time: 3–11 minutes.

End: Inhale deeply, hold your breath for 10 to 20 seconds, exhale. Repeat two more times, then relax.

COMMENTS: This Medical Meditation will help to dispel all of the old wounds, fears, and anger from the past, expecially your childhood, that you may still harbor in your first chakra. It will change you inside and out and help you to live in the present, magical moment.

MEDICAL MEDITATION FOR GENERATING HEALING ENERGY

Tune in and center yourself by chanting "Ong Namo, Guru Dev Namo" 3 times (Tune on page 143).

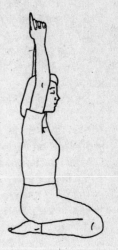

1. Posture: Sit in Rock Pose (see page 98 for reference) on your heels with your spine straight. You may also sit in a chair with your spine straight.

Focus: With your eyes closed, visualize a beam of light coming in at your navel point as you chant "Sat" and pull it in, and visualize the beam of light coming out of your third-eye point as you chant "Nam" and relax the navel.

Breath: The breath will come automatically as you chant.

Mantra: "Sat Nam" (rhymes with "but mom"). As you chant "Sat," apply the root lock (see page 88 for reference). As you chant "Nam," relax the lock. Do this in a consistent rhythm of approximately 8 to 10 times per 10 seconds.

Meaning of mantra: "My true identity."

Mudra: Interlace the fingers of both hands together with the index fingers pressed together and pointing straight up.

Time: 3–11 minutes. If you are a beginner you may start with 1 minute and gradually build up.

End: Inhale deeply, hold your breath for 10–15 seconds, and perfect your posture. Apply the root lock while holding the breath in. Exhale completely. Repeat 2 more times. On the last exhalation, hold the air out and apply the great lock. Focus on moving the energy up your spine to the top of your head, mentally channeling the energy to flow up to the top of the skull. Then rest for the same length of time you practiced this exercise.

COMMENTS: This Medical Meditation is called Sat Kriya, and it is one of the most powerful kriyas in the science of kundalini yoga. With regular practice, it increases lung capacity, perfects the functioning of the organs, stimulates circulation, generates great energy, and raises the kundalini energy up the spine.

I practice it daily for at least 3 minutes, and frequently prescribe it to patients. At 11 minutes, it is a complete kriya. During advanced white tantric yoga, it can be done for 31 minutes to 3 hours. In fact, I know practitioners who have done Sat Kriya for 2-1/2 hours a day for 40 days. This takes people to a whole new level of energy.

EASY MEDICAL MEDITATION FOR ENERGY

Tune in and center yourself by chanting "Ong Namo, Guru Dev Namo" 3 times (Tune on page 143).

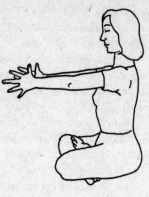

Posture: Sit in Easy Pose or in a chair with your back straight. Stretch your arms out in front of you, parallel to the ground, with your fingers wide apart and your palms facing each other.

Focus: The eyes are closed and focused at the third-eye point.

Breath: Long, deep and powerful breathing through the nose.

Mantra: Mentally repeat "Sat" on the inhale and "Nam" on the exhale.

Meaning of mantra: "My true identity."

Mudra: Same as posture.

Time: 3–11 minutes.

End: Inhale deeply, hold your breath, make fists of your hands, and slowly bring the fists to your chest with maximum tension. Slowly exhale when your fists touch your chest. Repeat 2 more times and then relax.

COMMENTS: This Medical Meditation improves vitality, endurance and productivity.

CHAPTER TWELVE

The Second Chakra

The Cradle of Creativity

A Case History

HEALING WITH THE SECOND CHAKRA

Maria, a thirty-two-year-old woman, first received a diagnosis of severe endometriosis in 1983, at age sixteen. Her physician at that time conducted extensive surgery to remove endometrial mass, and scar tissue.

At approximately this same time, Maria became deeply interested in meditation, and eventually became a professional spiritual counselor. Over a number of years, she honed the acumen of her intuition and psyche, and appeared to develop advanced abilities.

In 1992 Maria suffered an apparent recurrence of endometriosis, which is considered to be a recurring and incurable condition. A manual pelvic examination revealed an extensive pelvic mass, and she was scheduled for further surgery.

In the period between diagnosis and surgery, Maria meditated fervently, focusing upon second-chakra meditations. During these meditations, she employed two types of visual imagery. The first was an image of Jesus applying white light to the damaged areas. The second was an image of herself holding the damaged areas in her hands in a nurturing way, and observing them returning to a healthy color, texture, and size.

Maria also engaged in several meditative sessions in which she focused solely upon uniting with divine energy, and feeling the pleasure and power created by this union.

Just prior to her scheduled surgery, an ultrasound was performed, and to her surgeon's astonishment, the mass had disappeared. The surgery was canceled.

Seven years later, in 1999, Maria suffered a further recurrence, and surgery was performed. During this surgery, the surgeon noted that one of her fallopian tubes had recently ruptured, but had not caused internal bleeding, a common and potentially dangerous occurrence. Maria believed that her use of frequent advanced meditation may have helped to prevent this complication.

The surgeon believed that the ruptured fallopian tube required removal, but left it intact because he had agreed not to remove it without further consulting with the patient.

After the surgery, the doctor recommended follow-up surgery to remove the fallopian tube, and recommended hormonal therapy in the interim. Maria declined hormonal therapy, but agreed to another surgery, to be performed at a later date.

Maria again began to energetically apply Medical Meditation to her condition, and reported a variety of reactions. Despite her difficult medical condition, she experienced feelings of serenity, feelings of safety, and sometimes feelings of exhilaration. At one point, during a second-chakra meditation, she experienced, as she described it, "Ancient memories of the eternity of life."

At a subsequent examination, the doctor found no apparent dysfunction in the previously injured fallopian tube. He recommended against any further surgeries. Maria currently reports feeling increasingly healthy, and has suffered no further ill effects from her condition.

My clinical opinion is that Medical Meditation was a superb adjunctive modality in this case. It apparently helped Maria to heal herself on at least two occasions, without invasive medical intervention. This case history is an excellent example of how helpful Medical Meditation can be as a supportive therapy, used in conjunction with a more conventional therapy. Without the mutually supportive combination of therapies, it is likely that neither therapy would have achieved its fullest healing potential.

The General Characteristics of the Second Chakra

At a recent seminar, Betty, a middle-aged female therapist, approached me during a break and asked, "Dr. Khalsa, how do you live with an open heart in this world?" She looked at me searchingly, with soft-focus gray-blue eyes that were partly hidden by her shoulder-length hair. Betty seemed to be quite sensitive, and I was guessing that she expected me to say something metaphysical, such as, "Stay focused on your third-eye center, and learn to live in the ether."

Instead, I said something that made her eyes grow wide with surprise.

I replied, "Have strong lower chakras."

Oh my! It was as if I'd said, "The way to have an open heart in this world is to drive a pickup and chew tobacco."

Betty seemed completely caught up in the notion of chakras as hierarchical status symbols, with the higher chakras being far more . . . reputable . . . than the lower ones. This is a common but ill-founded perspective. There is nothing inherently substandard about the lower triangle of chakras. The lower chakras are, of course, more distanced from spirituality than the highest chakras. But without the lower chakras, we could never get to the higher chakras. Your first three chakras are your foundation, and without a strong foundation, you will suffer when the winds of change shift.

The second chakra is particularly important, and worthy of respect, because it is the virtual cornerstone of your foundation. As the heart and soul of your creativity, it sets the direction of all that follows it, including the actions of the higher, more esoteric chakras.

The second chakra, which extends from the top of the pelvic bone to the navel, is popularly perceived of as the sex chakra. But sexuality is mere metaphor for the power that resides here. The most fundamental characteristic of the second chakra—or *swadhistana,* in the Sanskrit—is its power to create and re-create, to give and receive. Ethereal healer Donna Eden, who can actually see the colors projected by chakras, has noted that in some people, their life color—the part of their auric field that does not change from birth to death—is the exact same color as their second chakra. This implies that the second chakra—in which lies the power of procreation—carries the force that survives us, even after death.

In fact, it is said that there are just three basic aspects of God: creation, organization, and destruction. Of these, creation is arguably the most sacred, as evidenced, in part, by the widespread appellation of God as the Creator. Thus, the second chakra is representative of one of the most revered aspects of being.

In our new, experience-centered Age of Aquarius, creativity is of heightened importance because we face a new world that demands creative new solutions to new problems. This need for creative solutions, I believe, is one reason why ever more people are turning to alternative medicine. The old ways just don't work, and alternative medicine grants us not just the condition of health, but also the experience of healing.

One reason the creative second chakra has the power to find new solutions is because it is characterized by the water element, the element that is mutable, fluid, ever-changing, and ever-flowing. Unlike the first chakra, which is associated with the earth element, the water element associated with the second chakra endows it with a profound sensibility of change. The ability to change, of course, is vital to good health, because the individual human body must at all times be able to respond to the constant cascade of changes that are sweeping through the universe.

On the physical level, the water element of the second chakra is mirrored by the secretions that emanate from the second chakra's glands and organs. The primary glands and organs of the second chakra include the penis, testicles, and prostate glands of males; the uterus, fallopian tubes, and vagina of females; and the kidneys and bladder. In addition, the second chakra helps govern the etheric energies of the adrenal glands (which are also influenced by the first chakra).

The flowing, mutable nature of the second chakra allows it to easily move its energies to other chakras, and also to the physical realm. Although the second chakra is very much a part of the noncognitive, nonintuitive lower triangle of chakras, it has a close relationship with the reflective sixth chakra, located at the third-eye point, or pituitary gland. The sixth chakra, the primary site of intuitive power, is absolutely reliant upon the creative energies of the second chakra. The second chakra empowers the sixth chakra with the passion that enables it to scale the heights of intuition. As Gurucharan says, "No chakra stands alone."

The freshness and newness that spring from the second chakra are reflected by the innocent, sweet nature that characterizes this chakra. Although many people think of the sexual urge as relentless and undiscriminating, this concept of sexuality reflects only the twisted, perverted sexuality that arises from frustration and hypersexual obsession. When allowed to flow naturally, the sexual urge—intimately bound to the procreative instinct—is open, innocent, and childlike. In fact, when some patients connect with their long-repressed second-chakra energies, they say that it is like connecting with their childhood self. There is a womblike element of total security connected with the second chakra, and this safe, secure feeling creates feelings of trust, generosity, and closeness.

Unlike the first chakra, which is focused almost solely upon selfhood, the second chakra needs the energies of others in order to flourish. On the most obvious level, it takes two people to procreate. On a deeper level, however, much of the creative instinct is involved with the reactions of others. Artists, writers, and musicians all generally have strong second-chakra energies, and they tend to feel unfulfilled if their creative work is not shared with and appreciated by others.

Thus, the second chakra allows our first experience of the merger of our selves with other selves, and with the universe. This merger is carried to its zenith by the sixth and seventh chakras—which merge spirit with spirit—but the first sweet taste of communion comes from the second chakra.

The merger of oneself with another person, through sex, long ago gave rise to the practice of tantric yoga, which is not well understood by the general public. Most people think that tantric yoga is concerned only with sexual union, but that type of yoga is confined solely to the practice of red tantric yoga. There are two other primary forms of tantric yoga. One is black tantric yoga, which involves mental manipulation, and the other is white tantric yoga, which involves spiritual connection, and cleansing of the subconscious. White tantric yoga can be quite illuminating, and has only one living master, my teacher, Yogi Bhajan.

Even though the spiritual union of white tantric yoga is more elevated than sexual union, sexual union can still be a mystical, spiritual experience, if energy is flowing freely between the second chakra and the fourth chakra: the heart chakra, the seat of compassion. In fact, one of the most wondrous capabilities of the second chakra is that of preparing the way for compassion. The second chakra endows the individual with the passion for attachment to another person, and this passion naturally ignites compassion, if energy is flowing freely.

The passion of the second chakra is the spark that sets fire to human desire. This desire may start as simple sexual energy, but the complexity of the human spirit transforms this primal sexual urge into a much broader, more variegated desire. For example, this phenomenon is expressed endlessly in the advertising that surrounds us. Probably the most repeated aphorism in the advertising profession is: Sex sells. Sexual images are used to sell everything from cars to cornflakes. The conventional wisdom is that people buy the advertised product in the hope that it will enhance their sexual attractiveness. But that's only part of why this advertising strategy is effective. In reality, most people are now too savvy to believe that an asexual product will somehow make them more sexually attractive. Instead, what they're responding to is the subliminal excitement of their generalized desire, which has been piqued by sexual imagery.

The sexual, creative energies that reside in the second chakra are most valuable and nurturing to the individual when the energy in the chakra is balanced, and allowed to flow freely in and out of the chakra. The same is true, of course, for the energies found in all chakras.

The energy that comes to the second chakra is carried primarily by the pingala nadi, the yang, active energy conduit associated with the right nostril. However, energy must also enter the second chakra from the ida nadi, the yin, passive energy conduit associated with the left nostril. If there is an imbalance in the proper ratio of ida/pingala energy entering the chakra, the energy in the chakra will become imbalanced. This is one reason why proper breathing is so important.

Imbalance, in this water-element chakra, will most often be manifested as isolation, if the chakra's energy is too weak, and as lust, if the chakra's energy is too strong. Both conditions are common in our society. Many people suffer from a weak second chakra, and lack passion and creativity. Their sex drive tends to be low, and they are prone to low energy. Many other people, though, suffer from an overactive second chakra, and become preoccupied with their sexuality. They tend to put sexual attraction at the top of their list of reasons for getting involved in relationships, but when this attraction wears off, they're left with nothing. These people may also be quite creative, but often burn out at a relatively early age.

The Physical Characteristics of the Second Chakra

From a physical perspective, when imbalance in the second chakra occurs, the organs that are most affected are the sex-related organs. The sex organs in both males and females are supplied with a rich vascular network and a powerful nerve plexus that arises from the lowest autonomic nerve plexus, the sacral plexus.

Therefore, long-term lack of energy in the second chakra sometimes results in impotence, and in impaired libido. There are several effective approaches to these problems, some of them of recent development.

Impotence is generally a devastating problem for men, because it not only robs them of an important, healthy source of pleasure but also often makes them feel unimportant in the larger sense, as human beings. The most widely known current treatment for organic impotence is the drug Viagra. In addition, effective treatment of vascular disorders is helping many men to regain sexual function. Also, approximately 20 percent of all impotence is due to psychological problems, such as depression, anger, and performance anxiety, which can be treated with counseling and medication. The most futuristic treatment for impotence is a microchip inserted near a major nerve in the scrotum, which stimulates the erectile response in reaction to arousal.

Impaired libido in males and females is also now effectively treated in many cases. The primary physiological treatment is hormone replacement therapy. Of particular value are the nonprescription hormones DHEA and pregnenolone, which millions of people have used to restore normal libidinal levels. These hormones help raise levels of testosterone, which is the prime mover of libido in males and females. Psychological factors are also a primary cause of low libido in many people, and can be ameliorated with counseling and medication.

Most of the causes of impotence and low libido can also be effectively treated, though, with Medical Meditation. This is often by far the best approach, because it does not entail the possible drug side effects, nor the expense of more conventional therapies. Medical Meditation successfully impacts the four major factors in impotence and libidinal dysfunction: vascular impairment, nervous system insufficiency, psychological problems, and hormonal imbalances. Medical Meditation, which of course includes yoga, restores blood flow, stimulates nervous system function, balances hormones (via the hypothalamic-pituitary axis), and helps to discharge psychological stressors.

Besides improving sexual function, Medical Meditation also enhances the general health of the sex organs. Thus it can help to prevent and alleviate problems such as prostate enlargement; prostatitis; uterine, cervical, prostate, and testicular cancer; and various gynecological problems.

Medical Meditation can also help mitigate many of the problems associated with menopause in women, such as fatigue, depression, low sex drive, insomnia, hot flashes, osteoporosis, and memory loss. Mood changes in female menopause can be markedly improved with Medical Meditation, especially if the meditation is performed as a part of one's regular program of sadhana. Many other discomforting symptoms of female menopause can be alleviated as well, by the normalizing of the hormonal profile.

Medical Meditation also helps males to resist the most invasive symptoms of male menopause, or age-associated hormonal decline, including depression, lethargy, insomnia, and reduced libido.

Medical Meditation is especially beneficial for both men and women if it is combined with a sensible lifestyle program of exercise, a low-fat diet with adequate protein, hormonal replacement therapy, herbal therapy, and food supplementation (with antioxidants, minerals, amino acids, and essential fatty acids).

The same restorative actions of Medical Meditation that improve the physical status of the sex-related organs and glands also nurture the physical health of the other organs and glands associated with the second chakra, including the kidneys, adrenals, and bladder. I have seen patients use Medical Meditation to help recover from kidney disorders, kidney disease, adrenal exhaustion, and urological problems.

Following are advanced meditations that will bring your second chakra to its highest state of function, and help you to solve real-world problems associated with energy imbalance in the second chakra.

Medical Meditations for the Second Chakra

SPECIAL MEDITATION FOR THE SECOND CHAKRA

Tune in and center yourself by chanting "Ong Namo, Guru Dev Namo" 3 times (Tune on page 143).

Posture: Sit in Easy Pose or in a chair with your spine straight.

Focus: Focus your eyes at the tip of your nose.

Breath: Inhale in the starting position, exhale as you bring your hands in and squeeze.

Mantra: Listen to the mantra "Ek Ong Kar Sat Gur Prasad" on tape.

Meaning of mantra: There is only one Creator who is realized by His grace.

Mudra: The hands are open with fingers straight.

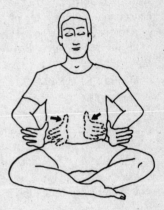

Begin by bringing your arms out to the sides, elbows bent, with the palms of the hands facing each other, about shoulder width apart. The hands are angled in toward each other at a 60-degree angle. Now bring your hands toward each other at the center of your body, but do not let them touch. This movement is strong and sharp, something like a clap without touching the hands. As your hands move inward, tighten the sex organ and release it as the hands move back to the starting position. For men, the tightening is centered at the base of the sex organ; for women, the contraction includes the clitoris. This is not a *mul bhanda;* the anus and navel point are not contracted with the sex organ.

Time: Begin with 11 minutes and slowly work up to 31 minutes.

End: Inhale and hold the breath, and tighten and tense every muscle in the body. Hold for 15 seconds and then relax. Repeat the cycle 2 more times.

COMMENTS: This Medical Meditation brings healing energy to ailments of the second chakra.

MEDICAL MEDITATION FOR MENSTRUAL REGULARITY

Tune in and center yourself by chanting "Ong Namo, Guru Dev Namo" 3 times (Tune on page 143).

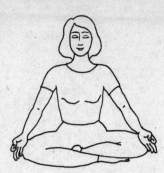

Posture: Sit in Easy Pose or in a chair with your spine straight. Relax your hands on your knees.

Focus: This is called the L-form of meditation. With each syllable you chant, visualize energy flowing in through the top of your head and out your third-eye point. The eyes are closed.

Breath: The breath will come automatically as you chant.

Mantra: "Sa Ta Na Ma."

Meaning of mantra: This mantra represents the cycle of creation. *Sa* means infinity; *Ta* means life; *Na* means death; *Ma* means rebirth.

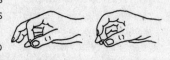

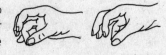

Mudra: On "Sa" touch the index finger to your thumb; on "Ta" touch the middle finger to your thumb; on "Na" touch the ring finger to your thumb; on "Ma" touch the little finger to your thumb. Apply a two-pound pressure every time you touch the fingers. Continue moving the fingers through the exercise, even during the silent part.

Time: 30 minutes total. Chant in a normal voice for 5 minutes, then whisper for 5 minutes, then go deep within yourself for 10 minutes (and still continue to repeat the mantra). Come back to the whisper for 5 minutes, and finally to the normal voice for 5 minutes.

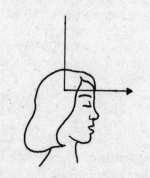

End: Inhale completely, then exhale all the air. Stretch the hands up as far as possible and spread them wide. Stretch the spine up and take several deep breaths.

COMMENTS: This Medical Meditation will help your body reestablish a menstrual rhythm after discontinuing the use of birth control pills. It also brings a very stable sense of mental balance.

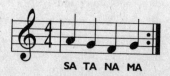

SA TA NA MA

The Third Chakra

Father Sun, Mother Earth

A Case History

HEALING WITH THE THIRD CHAKRA

Jayne, a forty-five-year-old female with a severely swollen liver, was told by her attending physician that she required a liver transplant. The doctor told her that if she did not replace her liver, which was twice its normal size, her death would be imminent.

Jayne accepted the idea of a liver transplant, but in the meantime sought a less invasive form of therapy. She was placed on a program of nutritional therapy and Medical Meditation. Jayne's nutritional therapy consisted of a diet of beets, daikon radishes, mung beans, and rice. Her Medical Meditations focused upon her third chakra, and specifically, of course, upon her liver.

In addition, a group of friends and healers performed a meditation called the Healing Ring of the Tantra on her behalf. This meditation is performed as follows: A group of eleven or more persons sits cross-legged in a circle, holding hands, eyes closed. The leader chants Wahe Guru, then the others in the group answer, Wahe Guru. Then the leader chants Sat Nam. The person to the left of the leader then becomes the leader, and the series of chants continues. The Healing Ring of the Tantra is used to generate nonlocal healing for a specific person. This meditation is to be done only on the new moon, full moon, or 11th day of the moon. The ring is never to be broken once it starts.

Jayne's liver soon stabilized on this program, and within three months it had become normal in size. The doctor's recommendation for a liver transplant was withdrawn. Jayne has since suffered no further problems with her liver.

Because Jayne's internist had been so adamant about the need for a transplant, I consider her recovery without the transplant to be extraordinary. I am convinced, with hindsight, that this recovery could not, in all probability, have occurred without the application of Medical Meditation. The liver is a particularly regenerative organ, and is easily influenced by naturalistic, regenerative modalities, including Medical Meditation. Jayne needed all the help she could get, and Medical Meditation was a significant and soothing contribution to her healing.

The General Characteristics of the Third Chakra

As we first enter life, life enters us through the umbilicus, and in those first few moments of human existence we begin to form the foundation of our own individual identity.

We age, we grow, we change, but throughout life our most primal, fundamental human identity remains situated in the place it began: in the umbilical area, surrounding the navel. This spot, the site of the third chakra, is the repository of each individual's own, special persona, and personal power.

The third chakra, located in the middle abdomen slightly below the tip of the sternum, is the physical location of the primary organs of digestion and assimilation—the stomach, intestines, liver, and pancreas—and it governs the energies of these organs. It also mirrors their function, on the ethereal plane. It is the chakra where nutritive ethereal energy is digested and dispersed to the 72,000 nadis—just as nutritive food energy is dispersed from the stomach.

The third chakra, or solar plexus chakra, is associated with the element of fire, and is often conceived of as a miniature sun, which helps burn food energy and radiate ethereal energy to the rest of the body. The solar plexus chakra is the chakra most involved with our sense of ego, ambition, fear, and fearlessness.

One apt metaphor for third-chakra activity is the description of ambition as fire in the belly. If the third chakra is overactive, it can create a hunger for power that can never be satisfied. In a sense, this fire in the belly can also burn a hole in the stomach—often quite literally, as an ulcer. If the chakra is underactive, however, it can create a sense of weakness, and an undeveloped sense of personal identity.

As the top chakra of the lower triangle of chakras, the third chakra is vitally important in enabling us to survive and succeed in the material world. Even though it sits atop the foundation of the chakra system (the lower three chakras), the third chakra is also in close communion with the higher chakras—particularly the fourth chakra, or heart chakra, and the sixth chakra, or third eye.

When functioning at its peak, the third chakra provides, as Dr. Gurucharan puts it, "the will of the spiritual warrior." As he notes, "The essence of a spiritual warrior is fearlessness, an ability to act with integrity, regardless of conditions." A person with a strong third chakra feels perpetually confident. It is almost as if this person's physical umbilical cord, at birth, were replaced by an ethereal umbilical cord, connecting the person to the power of the universe. To this person, the world is a nurturing entity, not the different world that is experienced by a person with a weak third chakra.

Because of this innate confidence, people with strong third chakras are rarely afraid to take action. They know that the quality of their life depends on the actions they take, and they aren't timid about taking the steps that are necessary to achieve the life they want. In contrast, people with weak solar plexus chakras, who don't really know who they are, often feel paralyzed by choice. They don't have a strong sense of self, so they don't know how to reflect their identity with their actions. Often, these people end up feeling like victims. They are tossed around by a world to which they're only weakly connected. These people are especially vulnerable to stress because stress often arises when a person feels out of control. Sometimes, people who feel like this try to overcompensate for their feelings of helplessness. They build elaborate systems of control around themselves, as a way to insulate themselves from the tempest-tossed world. They also try hard to control other people. A general principle of life is that people who don't feel in control of their own lives often try to control the lives of others.

This same obsession with control, however, is often shared by people who have overactive third chakras. If energy becomes trapped in the third chakra, causing a person to fixate there, they often become voracious for power. Unfortunately, though, this overabundance of energy in the third chakra creates a hunger for power that can never be satisfied. No matter how much power these people acquire, they always want more. As a rule, they base all their relationships around a power/submission differential.

Partly because the first energy to enter through the navel area was the energy of the mother, the third chakra is closely associated with parental sensibilities. The expectations of our parents are often lodged in our third chakra. This can cause a great deal of tension and pain, if there is a significant difference between what our parents want us to be and what we want to be.

This tension is heightened if there is a weak flow of energy between the second chakra and the third chakra. Our second chakra, as you'll recall, is our creative, child-focused chakra. If the child in us does not flow freely into our adult identity, as manifested by the third chakra, we will always feel frustrated and victimized. People with this problem often feel as if their lives consist of nothing but responsibility, commitment, and drudgery. To feel whole, and fully in control of our own lives, we must be in intimate contact with the inner child energy of the second chakra.

In adult life, though, it can be hard to get past the traumatic memories from childhood that suppress the flow of energy from the second chakra to the third. These memories, often seated in the subconscious, contribute to the isolation of the third chakra and the stagnation of its energies. However, Medical Meditations, especially those utilizing Breath of Fire and Sat Kriya, are especially valuable at unveiling long-hidden memories and dispelling them. When this happens, the energy flow between the second and third chakras is enhanced.

This energy, though, should not stay in the third chakra, but should circulate freely to the fourth chakra, and beyond. If the psychic energy of the past stays bottled up in the lower triangle of chakras, old wounds will stay fresh. People who suffer from this condition often act out their childhood traumas, in immature, inappropriate behaviors. For example, because they are afraid of change, they may create the same negative relationships over and over again, or remain in a job that is unsatisfying.

It's especially important that the feelings and energies of the third chakra should be transported to the cerebral sixth chakra, located behind the forehead. The reflective, highly cognitive sixth chakra area will make sense of the highly personal feelings found in the third chakra. The third-chakra feelings are likely to be narrowly centered around the needs of the ego, and around fear and personal power. However, the feelings of the sixth chakra—leavened with the compassion of the fourth chakra and the truth of the fifth chakra—are far more likely to encompass a broader vision of reality.

When the merging of energies with the other chakras occurs, the power of the third chakra achieves its highest function: the empowerment of the whole, integrated individual.

Physical Characteristics of the Third Chakra

On a physical level, the third chakra is most closely associated with the functions of the midabdominal glands and organs. In addition to the stomach, liver, and pancreas, these include the spleen, the gallbladder, the small intestine, some of the large intestine, the kidneys, and the adrenals. Some of these physical structures are also associated with the other chakras of the lower triangle. For example, the kidneys and adrenals are also influenced by energies emanating from the second chakra, and the large intestine is primarily influenced by the first chakra. Just as no chakra stands alone, neither does any organ nor gland. All organs and glands are linked, and are ultimately dependent not only upon one another but also upon the entire ethereal energy system.

The nervous system serves the abdominal organs primarily through the hypogastric and celiac nerve plexuses. The hypogastric plexus serves many of the upper intestinal organs and the stomach. The celiac plexus serves some of the midintestinal organs and the lower intestines. These plexuses also have branches that serve the kidneys, the adrenals, and other abdominal organs. Therefore, due to this rich nexus of nerve connections, it is eminently possible to influence third-chakra glands and organs by enhancing the ethereal energy flow of the third chakra. Nerve plexuses are gateways to chakras, and vice versa.

When the ethereal energy of the third chakra is flowing freely, the function of the digestive system is improved. This can result in amelioration of such conditions as hyperacid stomach, gastroesophageal reflux, stomach and duodenal ulcers, indigestion, food allergies and sensitivities, irritable bowel syndrome, and malabsorption syndrome. In addition, when digestion is improved, the function of the entire human body can be improved, since digestion provides the nutrients that fuel the body.

Other conditions involving third-chakra organs can also be alleviated, as well as prevented. These may include hepatitis B, hepatitis C, cirrhosis of the liver, gallstone formation, fatty liver, pancreatitis, diabetes, swelling of the spleen, and cancers of the liver, pancreas, and stomach.

One essential result of Medical Meditation upon the internal abdominal organs is increased blood flow. Of special value are certain kriyas that include kundalini yoga exercises, such as Sat Kriya, because these exercises flush the blood from the liver and pancreas and send it back to the heart. This not only cleanses and revitalizes these organs but also acts as a form of internal massage.

The third chakra, partly because of its close relationship with the sixth chakra, is also secondarily related to the eyes. In a metaphoric sense, the ability to see gives us a sense of control, and the third chakra is closely aligned with issues dealing with control.

Failure to establish a healthy sense of self, or integrated ego, is associated with the third chakra. On the most benign level, this may manifest as low self-esteem, and at the most pathological level, as borderline personality disorder, an extreme condition characterized by an almost complete lack of sense of self.

Particular negative emotions are associated with certain of the internal abdominal organs. The liver is associated with anger, owing perhaps to its function as the body's primary organ of detoxification, since toxicity often causes feelings of malaise and aggression. The kidneys are closely associated with fear. This may be partly due to the fact that the adrenal glands, which govern the stress response, are located adjacent to the kidneys. If these organs are not sufficiently nourished with ethereal energy, they may give rise to these emotions.

Following are various Medical Meditations and kundalini yoga exercises that enhance the function of the third chakra, and thereby improve the health of third-chakra organs and glands.

Medical Meditations for the Third Chakra

SPECIAL MEDITATION FOR THE THIRD CHAKRA

Tune in and center yourself by chanting "Ong Namo, Guru Dev Namo" 3 times (Tune on page 143).

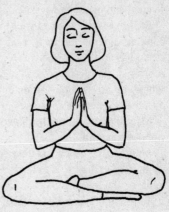

Posture: Sit in Easy Pose or in a chair with your spine straight.

Focus: Focus your eyes at the tip of your nose.

Breath: The breath will come automatically as you chant.

Mantra: This meditation is done to the mantra "Hummee Hum, Brahm Hum." The chanting is done with the tip of the tongue.

Meaning of mantra: "We are we, and we are one." On a higher spiritual level, it means we are already everything we need to be.

Mudra: Bend your elbows and bring your hands into prayer pose. All parts of the palms are touching and pressing together with equal force. Every time you chant "Hummee, Hum, Brahm, Hum," press your hands together, pull the navel in, and then release. Make sure you chant each word with the tip of the tongue. The hand press is a compression like the beat of the heart.

Time: 11 minutes.

End: Inhale and hold the breath, pull in on your navel, and press the tip of your tongue against the roof of your mouth. Hold for 15 seconds and exhale. Repeat the inhaling, holding the breath, pulling on your navel, pressing the tip of your tongue against the roof of the mouth, and exhaling 2 more times.

COMMENTS: When this Medical Meditation has been perfected, it may be practiced with the root lock instead of just the navel.

MEDICAL MEDITATION TO IMPROVE DIGESTION

Tune in and center yourself by chanting "Ong Namo, Guru Dev Namo" 3 times
(Tune on page 143).

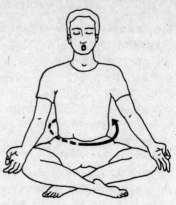

Posture: Sit in Easy Pose or in a chair with
your spine straight and chin in.

Focus: With your eyes closed, focus on
sending energy to the navel point.

Breath: Make a beak of your mouth and
drink air through the beak. Hold the air in
as long as possible as you churn your stomach around and around. When you must
exhale, do so through the mouth without
pressure.

Mantra: This Medical Meditation is done
without a mantra.

Mudra: The hands are relaxed on the
knees in gyan mudra, with the index fingers
touching the thumbs.

Time: Do this exercise a total of 3 times at one sitting.

End: Inhale through the mouth, hold your breath for 5–10 seconds, exhale
through the mouth, and relax.

COMMENTS: This Medical Meditation is also called Vatskar Dhouti Kriya, and
should only be done on an empty stomach. If you are doing other exercises, make
this the last exercise in the series. After this Medical Meditation drink 2 quarts of
water and avoid hot, spicy foods for the rest of the day.

Vatskar Dhouti Kriya is said to help eliminate all digestive problems, including
chronic excess acidity. Since many other diseases, such as colds and flu, can start
with problems of digestion and elimination, this kriya works toward general health
as well.

NOTES ON DIGESTION: You cannot digest food properly unless you schedule relaxation into your days. You also need mild daily activity, such as walking, to keep
your body strong and healthy, and to massage the organs of digestion and elimination. During the day, take a 10-minute nap or rest after eating. In the evening,
take a walk after your meal. This will stimulate your digestive system, so that when
you sleep, your body can be totally at rest, not diverting energy to the digestive
process.

MEDICAL MEDITATION TO CLEANSE THE LIVER

Tune in and center yourself by chanting "Ong Namo Guru Dev Namo" 3 times (Tune on page 143).

Posture: Sit in Easy Pose or in a chair with your back straight. Make wide circles with your torso by grinding at the waist. First rotate in one direction, then switch direction.

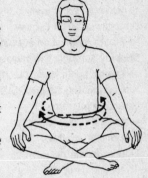

Focus: The eyes are closed and focused at the third-eye point. Also, visualize sending healing energy to your liver.

Breath: Inhale during the backward semi-circle, exhale as you circle forward.

Mantra: This Medical Meditation is done without a mantra.

Mudra: Hold your knees with your hands, and use this as a pull/push tool while making the circles.

Time: 1–2 minutes per direction.

End: Inhale in the center, hold your breath for 10–30 seconds. Exhale and relax.

MEDICAL MEDITATION FOR THE GALLBLADDER

Tune in and center yourself by chanting "Ong Namo, Guru Dev Namo" 3 times (Tune on page 143).

Posture: Lie on your back. Place your right hand under the small of your back, palm down. Place your left palm against the back of your neck, elbow touching the floor. Raise your right leg to 90 degrees.

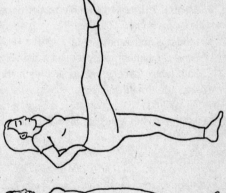

Focus: With your eyes closed, focus on sending energy to the gallbladder.

Breath: Do Breath of Fire when the right leg is up.

Mantra: This Medical Meditation is done without a mantra.

Mudra: Same as posture.

Time: 1–3 minutes.

End: Inhale completely and hold the breath for 15 seconds. Exhale and relax down into Corpse Pose (see page 99 for reference). Deeply relax for 1–3 minutes.

COMMENTS: This Medical Meditation is useful in correcting problems of the gallbladder, heart, and spleen.

MEDICAL MEDITATION TO STRENGTHEN THE PANCREAS

Tune in and center yourself by chanting "Ong Namo, Guru Dev Namo" 3 times (Tune on page 143).

1. Posture: Kneel in Rock Pose, sitting on your heels (see page 98 for reference). Cross your hands over your navel and bring your forehead to the floor and your buttocks up to 60 degrees.

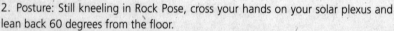

Focus: With your eyes closed, focus on sending energy to the pancreas.

Breath: Long, slow, deep breathing.

Mantra: This Medical Meditation is done without a mantra.

Mudra: Same as posture.

Time: 3 minutes.

End: Inhale deeply, hold your breath for 10 seconds, exhale.

2. Posture: Still kneeling in Rock Pose, cross your hands on your solar plexus and lean back 60 degrees from the floor.

Focus: With your eyes closed, focus on sending energy to the pancreas.

Breath: Long, slow, deep breathing.

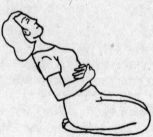

Mantra: This Medical Meditation is done without a mantra.

Mudra: Same as posture.

Time: 3 minutes.

End: Inhale deeply, hold your breath for 10 seconds, exhale and relax.

COMMENTS: This Medical Meditation helps control blood sugar.

MEDICAL MEDITATION FOR THE KIDNEYS

Tune in and center yourself by chanting "Ong Namo, Guru Dev Namo" 3 times (Tune on page 143)

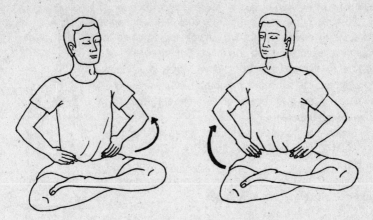

Posture: Sit in Easy Pose or in a chair with your spine straight. Place your hands on your waist. Twist your torso left and right, combining it with the breath.

Focus: The eyes are closed and focused to the third-eye point.

Breath: All breathing is done through your nose. Inhale as you twist to the left, exhale as you twist to the right.

Mantra: Mentally repeat Sat on the inhale, and Nam on the exhale.

Meaning of mantra: My true identity.

Mudra: Same as posture.

Time: 1–5 minutes.

End: Inhale deeply in the center, hold your breath for 10 seconds, exhale, and relax.

COMMENTS: This Medical Meditation optimizes kidney function.

MEDICAL MEDITATION FOR THE LOWER TRIANGLE OF CHAKRAS
(TO REPAIR STRESS DAMAGE)

Tune in and center yourself by chanting "Ong Namo, Guru Dev Namo" 3 times
(Tune on page 143).

Posture: Sit in Easy Pose or in a chair with your spine
straight. Extend your right arm straight up, hugging the
right ear. Extend your left arm up at 60 degrees from horizontal, with the palm facing down. Press your elbows
straight and stretch your arms up from your shoulders.

Focus: Keep your eyes slightly open, and look down
toward the upper lip.

Breath: Long, slow, deep breathing through the nose.

Mantra: This Medical Meditation is done without a
mantra.

Mudra: On both hands, put your thumb onto the
mound just below your little finger.

Time: 3–11 minutes.

COMMENTS: This Medical Meditation alleviates any problem in the lower spine. It
is a direct healer for the kidneys and adrenal glands. Consequently, it helps repair
the energy drained by long-term stress. This kriya also helps the heart. You will find
that the breath will automatically become longer and deeper as you continue. It is
important to hold the arms perfectly still to receive full benefit.

CHAPTER FOURTEEN

The Fourth Chakra

From Passion to Compassion

A Case History

HEALING WITH THE FOURTH CHAKRA

John, a male in his fifties, was first diagnosed with advanced emphysema in the mid-1980s, and was given a prognosis of approximately two years to live. John had previously suffered from asthma and had smoked, but had stopped smoking four years prior to onset of his emphysema symptoms, which included extreme shortness of breath, a heavy feeling in his chest, and fatigue.

John was immediately placed upon a program of Medical Meditation, as well as appropriate medications. The medications were intended to reduce symptoms, not to reverse the course of the disease; emphysema is almost universally considered to be irreversible.

John had previously been exposed to yoga, but later stated that he had thought yoga is for sissies. His meditations focused primarily upon the fourth chakra, with a number of pranayama breathing exercises. John practiced his Medical Meditations assiduously, and as his symptoms began to ameliorate, he reduced his reliance upon medication.

Within five years John had eliminated use of medication. A breathing test was performed, and it was determined that his lung capacity was 49 percent below normal. For John, that was an improvement upon previous tests, in spite of the fact that emphysema is invariably considered to be progressively debilitating. John continued his Medical Meditations and also became quite interested in spiritual literature, in response to his apparent improvement.

John's breathing capacity continued to improve. He began to perform yoga breathing exercises even better than most of his fellow yoga students.

John gradually lost interest in medical evaluations of his condition, preferring to trust his own perception of his improving health. However, seven years after his last medical breathing test, he took another one, in order to qualify for an insurance policy. This test indicated that he had 98 percent of the normal breathing capability of a man his age.

John's remarkable recovery has since been maintained. He has no significant functional symptoms of the emphysema that once threatened his life.

The General Characteristics of the Fourth Chakra

For many centuries, among a multitude of cultures, love was thought to live in the heart. With the advent of modern anatomy, though, scientists came to believe that love, like all other emotions, resided solely in the brain.

Today, however, we've come full circle. In our current era of what might be called postmodern anatomy, the new medical perspective recognizes the ethereal body as well as the physical body. Physicians who treat the ethereal body now see that there is, indeed, an inseparable connection between love and the heart.

One of the most fascinating indications of the link between emotions and the heart recently emerged from data collected in the treatment of heart transplant patients. In a significant number of cases, patients who received a transplanted heart also seemed to inherit some of the most basic likes and dislikes of their deceased heart donors. Some found themselves, for example, suddenly and inexplicably liking the foods and colors that their heart donor had liked.

This anecdotal evidence, though, is less compelling than the simple evidence that lies within your own experience. The link between your own heart and your emotions is almost certainly something you have felt many times. For example, when you have felt deep stirrings of love for someone, you probably experienced a sense of expansiveness in your chest. Or during grief, when you felt as if your heart were breaking, you may have felt a heaviness in your chest, or even a dull ache in your heart.

Even the latest research on brain peptides has shown that the link between love and the heart is more than mere metaphor. The brain's peptides, as I indicated in earlier chapters, are not located strictly in the brain, as long believed. Instead, these proteinlike molecules of emotion and molecules of information are dispersed throughout the body, and are particularly prevalent in certain organs, including the gut and the heart. For example, we now know that certain neuropeptides that govern heart rate are found in the heart itself. This indicates that the heart, to some degree, does its own thinking about how fast to beat.

Furthermore, this self-decided heart rate can even influence the frequency of brain waves, through the principle of entrainment. Entrainment, as I discussed in the chapter on sound, is the tendency of one pulsating entity to copy the rhythm of a stronger entity, as when a small metronome naturally adheres to the beat of a larger one. The electrical wave produced by a heartbeat has fifty times the amplitude of a brain wave, and a thousand times as much strength. Thus, the heart has at least some capacity to make the brain follow the rhythms of the heart. For example, the heart can change fast, stressful beta brain waves into calming alpha waves.

However, to be strictly accurate, according to the tenets of postmodern anatomy, it is not just the heart that is so laden with intelligence and esoteric power: it is the fourth chakra, in which the heart lies. The fourth chakra, or heart chakra, is not only the site of the physical heart but also the site of one of the body's most exquisite centers of ethereal energy. Many of the qualities that are ascribed to the heart, such as love or courage, may well be in the heart, since the heart is in the fourth chakra, but they are not of the heart: they are the qualities of the fourth chakra.

The fourth chakra is often described as a transitional chakra, because it makes the transition between the lower triangle of chakras and the upper triangle. The symbol for the fourth chakra, therefore, is the familiar six-pointed Star of David, which is formed by two triangles overlapping each other. The fourth chakra is the connecting point for the lower chakras' self-absorbed, survival-oriented qualities, and the higher chakras' spiritual, other-directed, outward-bound qualities. Because of its elevated ethereal qualities, the fourth chakra is associated with the element of air. The fourth chakra also has a literal association with the air element, because the lungs lie in the fourth chakra.

The lower three chakras are involved mostly in the mastering of human impulses. The fourth chakra, though, has a more elevated, esoteric level of function. When your heart chakra opens and receives energy from the lower triangle, it endows you with your deepest appreciation of other people. No longer is your self-awareness limited to just your own perspective. Now you can see yourself through the eyes of others. No longer do you feel isolated and alone. Now you can share your selfhood with others, through the communion that we call love. Because of this extraordinary quality of expansiveness, the fourth chakra spreads a person's concern from me to we.

When you are able to truly feel the existence of others, it changes your own primal view of your selfhood. It expands it. The dividing lines between me and we begin to blur, until finally you begin to see that the distinctions separating them are, on the ethereal plane, artificial: Me is we.

When you reach this state of expanded awareness, it profoundly blesses your life. It blesses you forever with a sense of companionship, no matter how alone you may be. It even blesses you with a sense of deathlessness because you stop identifying your life as just your own physical, personal selfhood.

When this state of personal transcendence occurs, it can free your soul from grief. It can allow you to finally put an end to the grief of loss: the loss of loved ones, the loss of the past, and the loss of your own life (a type of grief that you experience as fear). As you begin at last to merge with the greater you that exists beyond the boundaries of body and time, you rise above the feelings of finiteness and aloneness that torture the people who are trapped in their lower chakras.

Conversely, though, too much grief can freeze the flow of energy entering the fourth chakra. When you've been hurt so badly that you feel you can never love again, you can turn this foreboding feeling into a self-fulfilling prophecy. This happens to many people. They lose a loved one, through divorce or death, and then, to protect their feelings, they focus too fully on just their lower-chakra obsession with survival. Often they throw themselves into their work and shut down their emotions. When this happens, they can endanger not just their spiritual lives but also their energy-starved, fourth-chakra organs. Grief is a killer. It depresses immunity terribly, partly by reducing the function of the fourth chakra's thymus. It also significantly contributes to heart disease. Contrary to conventional wisdom, grief can be as hard on the heart as the stress caused by anger.

When your fourth chakra is activated by free-flowing energy, though, it can help you overcome grief, by bringing you closer to the spiritually evolved condition known as the neutral mind. The neutral mind does not label things with polarized qualities, such as good and bad, or loss and gain. Instead, it accepts all things, and makes no judgments. When your fourth chakra is open, and your neutral mind is fully awake, you love without attachment, you love without judgment, and you love without even the expectation of being loved in return. The neutral mind has a powerful sense of inclusion, expansion, and belonging. It is strong enough to overcome any sense of loss or separation. Having a vibrantly strong neutral mind is one of the best possible ways to avoid depression or obsession.

The neutral mind and the open heart allow us to connect with not just other people but actually reality. Unfortunately, many people are so wrapped up in their isolation and fear that they cannot, as the expression goes, see what's right in front of them. Nor can they express true, unvarnished reality, as upward-bound energy moves on to the next chakra, the throat chakra. As Yogi Bhajan has remarked, "A truth spoken in fear is a lie."

When the fourth chakra widens our perspective, connects us to others, and brings us closer to reality, it plants the seed of intuition. Intuition comes to full flower in the sixth chakra, located near the forehead, but without the fourth chakra, there can be no intuitiveness. In fact, the fourth chakra is the first gate to the subconscious. On many occasions, I've noticed that when my fourth chakra is open, I am better able to remember my dreams, and to grasp their meaning.

When we open the fourth chakra, though, and lay bare our hearts, we are bound to get hurt. There can be no pleasure without pain, and no joy without sorrow. These are the polarities that swirl the energies of the fourth chakra and increase its strength.

Often, the pain that you may feel when you open your heart chakra is pain from your past. Sometimes, during Medical Meditation, your remembrances of past pain may be so vivid that you will feel as if you are reliving them. You must grapple with these painful memories, though, to truly heal. Aided by the widened perspective and the compassion of your fourth chakra, you will be able to see these past events with new eyes—eyes that will allow you to look past your own personal hurts and the anger and fear these hurts caused. When this happens, you'll be able to view with compassion events that you once saw only with passion.

When people begin this process, they often feel as if their loftiest possible goal will be to find a way to forgive the people who hurt them. But almost all people eventually find—as did I, myself—that the person who has hurt them the most, for the longest time, is the person they least suspected: themselves.

In all likelihood, no one has pushed you as hard, denied you pleasure as often, nor held you in contempt as much as you have yourself. Too often, for too long, you have been your own worst enemy. I'm sure you can remember many of the occasions when this has occurred. For you to completely heal, even your worst enemy must be forgiven.

Only through this pivotal self-forgiveness can you ever reach the greatest achievement of selfhood: love of your self. True love of self is not narcissistic, nor is it even self-centered. Those traits are nothing but the contrived window-dressing of self-hate. True love of self is simple acceptance. Without it, you can never be happy, nor even fully healthy. Without it, you can never love others. This is the ultimate lesson of the fourth chakra.

The Physical Characteristics of the Fourth Chakra

The primary organ of the fourth chakra is the heart, but the lungs and the thymus gland are also vitally important. Of course, these three physical structures work in close concert. The lungs furnish the heart's blood with oxygen, and the thymus supplies the blood with the immune substances the body needs to fight disease.

The most common diseases associated with dysfunction of the fourth chakra's organs and glands are: high blood pressure; coronary artery disease; arteriosclerosis; asthma; chronic obstructive lung disease; autoimmune disorders such as lupus, rheumatoid arthritis, and polymyositis; and cancer, which is essentially an immune-dysfunction disease.

The primary innervation of the fourth chakra organs comes from the largest single nerve in the body, the vagus nerve. The vagus nerve, or wandering nerve, is the tenth cranial nerve, and exits the brain from the brain stem. It travels through an opening, or foramen, that is close to the jawbone and serves many of the organs of the upper chest, including the heart, stomach, and esophagus. Because the vagus nerve travels through the jaw area, it is especially sensitive to stimulation from vibratory chanting.

In addition, the cardiac plexus, from the sympathetic branch of the autonomic nervous system, sends multiple nerves to the heart, to the largest blood vessels, and to the lungs. As you probably remember, the autonomic nervous system is the part of the nervous system that is not actively governed by thought, but instead is automatic. It consists of the speed-up sympathetic branch, and the slow-down parasympathetic branch. Because the autonomic nervous system is such an integral part of the nerve supply to the fourth chakra organs, it is important that the autonomic nervous system remain balanced between its sympathetic and parasympathetic branches. As I've shown, one of the best ways to balance the autonomic nervous system is with Medical Meditation. If imbalance occurs, it can result in a variety of disorders. For example, sympathetic dominance can contribute to high blood pressure, and parasympathetic dominance can contribute to a slow pulse. The lungs are also often affected by autonomic nervous system imbalance, even though some physicians underestimate this effect. Stress, for example, is well known to cause bronchioconstriction and asthma, while meditation can help relax the bronchi.

One of the most striking effects of Medical Meditation upon fourth-chakra organs is its ability to help prevent heart disease. As demonstrated previously, regular meditators have markedly lower incidence of heart disease than nonmeditators. The major risk factors for heart disease are smoking, being overweight, having untreated high blood pressure, being sedentary, and experiencing unbalanced stress. Every one of these risk factors is reduced by Medical Meditation. Smoking and overeating almost invariably diminish when people begin to meditate, as does the tendency to be sedentary. Furthermore, meditation reduces blood pressure, and alleviates stress. At one clinic in which I used Medical Meditation, we achieved an extraordinary 75 percent success rate among patients who were trying to stop smoking.

A secondary cardiovascular benefit of Medical Meditation is its ability to reduce use of antihypertensive medications, which can have negative side effects. Harvard's Dr. Herbert Benson has demonstrated convincingly that when patients begin to meditate, they can reduce and even eliminate use of drugs for high blood pressure.

Medical Meditation also has a profound effect upon the behavioral characteristics that contribute to cardiovascular disease. Certain personality types appear to be more prone to heart attacks, particularly hard-driving, type-A people who hold in a lot of repressed anger. One recent study showed that 15 percent of doctors and lawyers with highly elevated hostility die by age fifty. It is believed that anger and tension kill primarily by destabilizing the balance of hormones, which raises blood pressure, stresses the heart, and decreases immunity. Similarly, depression also has a markedly negative effect upon the heart. Some researchers now believe that depression is as stressful to the cardiovascular system as anger and hostility. Some of the world's most prominent cardiovascular specialists, including Dr. Dean Ornish, have proven that meditation markedly improves the personality traits, whether agitated or depressed, that contribute to heart disease. Another fourth-chakra disease that is powerfully impacted by Medical Meditation is asthma. Bronchial spasms can be made worse by stress, and Medical Meditation is one of the best countermeasures against stress. Furthermore, the pranayama breathing exercises of Medical Meditation are excellent for people with asthma. As an asthmatic child, I experienced the importance of breathing exercises myself. My uncle, an esteemed cardiologist, prescribed a series of breathing exercises for me that helped immensely. Even so, my lungs remained somewhat weak, and I was prone to bronchitis and even bronchial spasm in my early adulthood. However, when I began to do Medical Meditation, with a strong focus on breathing exercises, my vulnerability to lung problems ceased.

The third major physical structure of the fourth chakra is the thymus. It has long been recognized that the thymus generally atrophies with age, and this is believed to partially account for the lower immunity experienced by many older people. However, it may well be that people who regularly meditate, and bring energy to the fourth chakra, do not experience this same decline. This might, in fact, account for the enhanced resistance to disease exhibited by regular meditators. As Richard Gerber, M.D., states in *Vibrational Medicine*, "It is possible that age-related involution of the thymus gland is not a universal phenomenon. In those who do have thymic atrophy in later years, there may be a relationship between loneliness, depression, blockage of the heart chakra, and loss of glandular function." Physicians have for many years known that depression and grief are primary depressors of immunity, and it may be that depression and grief decrease the activity of the thymus by blocking energy to the fourth chakra.

Improvement of thymus gland function not only increases resistance to disease but also decreases vulnerability to autoimmune disorders, in which the immune system turns against the body. The most common autoimmune disease is rheumatoid arthritis. Others include lupus and polymyositis. When these diseases occur, the body is essentially incapable of telling the difference between an invading organism and the body itself. In effect, it fails to distinguish between self and nonself. On the ethereal level, this represents a failure of a vital fourth-chakra function: the ability to accept one's self, and to recognize the difference between self and others, without feeling threatened, and then overreacting.

As you can see, the consequences of dysfunction in the fourth chakra can be dire. The fourth chakra is a pivotal energy center, the doorway to the higher energy centers, and the site of the organs that bring the blood of life and the breath of life. Following are Medical Meditations that improve fourth-chakra function.

Medical Meditations for the Fourth Chakra

SPECIAL MEDITATION FOR THE FOURTH CHAKRA

Tune in and center yourself by chanting "Ong Namo, Guru Dev Namo" 3 times (Tune on page 143).

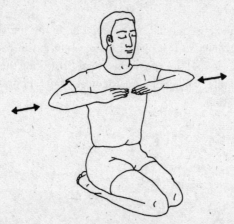

Posture: Sit in Rock Pose on your heels or in a chair with your spine straight. The starting position is with your upper arms parallel to the ground, on the same level as your shoulders. Your elbows are bent, and your fingertips are nearly touching each other at the center of your chest near your heart center. From the starting position, your hands and forearms move out to the sides, palms facing down. Pull your navel point in strongly and lift your solar plexus and diaphragm slightly in a focused motion. As your arms move back in, your navel is released. Continue this movement in rhythm with the music.

Focus: Your eyes are focused at the tip of your nose.

Breath: The breath is coordinated with the movement. Inhale as you relax the navel, exhale as you pull the navel in. All breathing is done through the nose.

Mantra: This Medical Meditation is done to the mantra "Hummee Hum, Brahm Hum," but the meditation is silent.

Meaning of mantra: "We are we, and we are one." On a higher spiritual level, it means we are already everything we need to be.

Mudra: The hands are flat with the palms facing downward.

Time: 11 minutes.

End: Inhale and hold your breath for 15 seconds and then release. Repeat two more times.

COMMENTS: This Medical Meditation opens the heart center.

MEDICAL MEDITATION FOR THE NEUTRAL MIND

Tune in and center yourself by chanting "Ong Namo, Guru Dev Namo" 3 times (Tune on page 143).

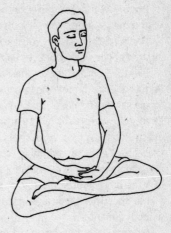

Posture: Sit in Easy Pose or in a chair with your spine straight. Remove all tension from every part of your body. Sit straight, with balance.

Focus: Close your eyes. Imagine seeing yourself sitting peacefully and full of radiance. Then gradually let your energy collect, like a flow, at the brow point.

Breath: Let your breath regulate itself in a slow, meditative manner. All breathing is done through the nose.

Mantra: Concentrate without effort and, at that point, mentally vibrate a simple monotone as if chopping the sound. Project each syllable distinctly: "Wha-hey gu-roo."

Meaning of mantra: This is the Mantra of Ecstasy; it means "Out of darkness, into light."

Mudra: Put both of your hands in your lap with the palms facing up. Put your right hand into the left. Your thumb tips may touch or not.

Time: 11 to 31 minutes.

COMMENTS: It is easy to hear a truth, but difficult to live it—imbed it deeply into your heart and mind. The Neutral Mind opens the gate to that deep remembrance of the self and soul. The Neutral Mind lives for the touch of vastness. It lets other thoughts be, without disturbing your inner light. Call on your higher self and keep going steadily through all barriers. Let it go and let it flow. See how the universe provides.

MEDICAL MEDITATION FOR A CALM HEART

Tune in and center yourself by chanting "Ong Namo, Guru Dev Namo" 3 times (Tune on page 143).

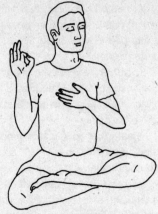

Posture: Sit in Easy Pose or in a chair with your spine straight.

Focus: Either close your eyes, or look straight ahead with your eyes half open.

Breath: Concentrate on the flow of breath. Regulate each bit of the breath consciously. Inhale slowly and deeply through both nostrils. Then hold your breath in by suspending your chest. Retain as long as possible. Then exhale through the nose smoothly, gradually, and completely. When your breath is totally out, lock the breath out for as long as possible.

Mantra: This Medical Meditation is done without a mantra.

Mudra: Place your left hand on the center of your chest at your heart center level. The palm is flat against your chest and your fingers are horizontal and pointing to the right. The right hand is in gyan mudra; that is, the index finger touches the thumb. The other fingers are straight. Raise your right hand to your right side as if giving a pledge. Your palm faces forward. Your elbow is relaxed near your side with your forearm perpendicular to the ground.

Time: 3–5 minutes.

End: Inhale and exhale strongly 3 times.

COMMENTS: The proper home of the subtle force of prana is in the lungs and heart. The left palm is placed at the natural home of the prana. Create a deep stillness at that point. The right hand that throws you into action and analysis, is placed in a receptive, relaxed mudra and put in the position of peace. The entire posture induces a feeling of calmness. This Medical Meditation technically creates a still point for the prana at the heart center.

Emotionally, it adds clear perception to your relationships with yourself and others. If you were upset at work or upset in a personal relationship, sit in this meditation for 3 to 5 minutes before deciding how to act. Then act with your full heart.

This is perfect for beginners. It opens your awareness of breath, and it conditions the lungs and heart. This is a very precious Medical Meditation.

MEDICAL MEDITATION FOR THE IMMUNE SYSTEM

Tune in and center yourself by chanting "Ong Namo, Guru Dev Namo" 3 times
(Tune on page 143).

Posture: Sit in Easy Pose or in a chair with your
spine straight.

Focus: The eyes are closed and focused at the
third-eye point.

Breath: Begin a steady, powerful Breath of Fire.
Emphasize the beat at your navel point.

Mantra: This Medical Meditation is done without
a mantra.

Mudra: Your left hand is at shoulder level, with
the left arm bent and forearm perpendicular to the
ground, and facing forward. Make surya mudra
with your left hand: touch the tip of your ring finger
to the tip of your thumb. Your right hand is in a fist,
with only the index finger extended. Close off your
right nostril with your right index finger.

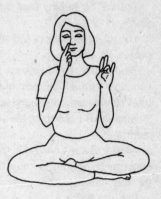

Time: 3 minutes.

End: Inhale and hold your breath. As you hold,
interlace your fingers and put your palms in front of
the thymus, just below the throat, about 4 inches
away. Try to pull your fingers apart. Resist and create
tension. When you must, exhale. Inhale, and hold
your breath and repeat the pulling three more times.

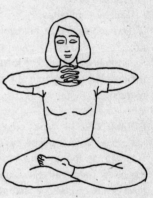

COMMENTS: The immune system interacts with the
central nervous system, the glands, and the emotions. We are each given the strength to encounter
life's challenges. We have moral strength, mental
strength, emotional strength, and physical strength. All these strengths are inter-
connected. We block the flow of that strength when we experience feelings of
anger, self-defeatism, and self-blame. To boost the immune system we must overcome these blocks.

The right hemisphere stores many of the diffuse negative emotions that lead us
to depression, and to a lower functioning immune system. This Medical Meditation helps the sympathetic system and the right hemisphere to adjust themselves.
Relax and keep going until you are through the emotional inertia. Then you will
feel light, energized, and hopeful.

With this Medical Meditation, the immune system will have new vigor, and will
not be blocked by inner conflict. This type of breathing is called the Sun Breath.

MEDICAL MEDITATION FOR HIGH BLOOD PRESSURE

Tune in and center yourself by chanting "Ong Namo, Guru Dev Namo" 3 times (Tune on page 143).

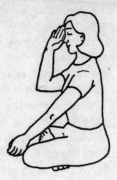

Posture: Sit in Easy Pose or in a chair with a straight spine.

Focus: The eyes are closed and focused at the third-eye point.

Breath: Use the thumb of your right hand to block your right nostril. Do Breath of Fire through your left nostril while pumping your navel point in and out.

Mantra: This Medical Meditation is done without a mantra.

Mudra: The left hand is in gyan mudra, with the index finger touching your thumb. The right thumb is blocking the right nostril, and the other fingers are together, pointing straight up.

Time: 1–3 minutes.

End: Inhale deeply, hold your breath for 10–20 seconds, exhale. Repeat 2 more times.

Contraindications: For long-standing problems of high blood pressure, do 10 minutes daily of normal left nostril breathing (without Breath of Fire or stomach pumping).

COMMENTS: The more completely you can pull your abdomen in and pull it out, the more effective will be this Medical Meditation.

Breathing through the left nostril stimulates the cooling, relaxing functions of the body. The breath flows mainly through only one nostril at any one time. The flow of breath switches naturally from one nostril to the other every 2 1/2 hours throughout the day. When you need to reduce tension, breathe through the left nostril.

MEDICAL MEDITATION TO PREVENT HEART ATTACKS

Tune in and center yourself by chanting "Ong Namo, Guru Dev Namo" 3 times (Tune on page 143).

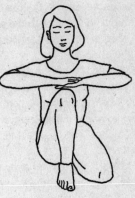

Posture: With a straight spine, sit with your left heel at the perineum (the area midway between the genitals and the anus). The right knee is at the chest, foot flat on the floor. Forearms are parallel to the floor.

Focus: Look down as deeply as possible.

Breath: Completely inhale in 4 equal sniffs. Exhale completely in 4 equal breaths through the nose.

Mantra: You may use any mantra you wish with the breath. A good one is "Ong, Ong, Ong, Ong" repeated mentally as you inhale, and "Sohung, Sohung, Sohung, Sohung" repeated mentally as you exhale.

Meaning of mantra: This is a heart opening and empowering mantra that means, "The Creator is within me."

Mudra: The hands are flat and facing down, with the right palm resting on top of the left hand; tips of thumbs are touching.

Time: 7 minutes. Add 5 minutes for each week of practice. You may work up to 31 minutes per session.

End: Inhale deeply, hold your breath for 10 seconds, exhale. Repeat 2 more times.

COMMENTS: According to ancient wisdom, this Medical Meditation keeps the heart arteries open.

MEDICAL MEDITATION FOR THE THYMUS GLAND

Tune in and center yourself by chanting "Ong Namo, Guru Dev Namo" 3 times (Tune on page 143).

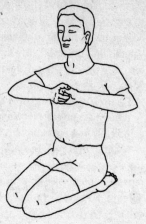

Posture: Sit in Rock Pose on your heels, or in Easy Pose, or in a chair with the spine straight.

Focus: The eyes are closed and focused at the third-eye point.

Breath: All breathing is done through the nose. Inhale, hold your breath, and without separating your hands, try to pull them apart. Apply maximum force. Exhale. Inhale and continue.

Mantra: This Medical Meditation is done without a mantra.

Mudra: Place your hands in bear grip at the heart level, keeping the arms parallel to the floor.

Time: 1–3 minutes.

End: Inhale deeply through the nose, hold for 5–10 seconds, exhale and relax.

COMMENTS: In this exercise you are resisting your own force. Besides stimulating the thymus gland, this Medical Meditation opens the heart center.

MEDICAL MEDITATION FOR STRESS RELIEF AND
RESOLVING ISSUES FROM THE PAST

Tune in and center yourself by chanting "Ong Namo, Guru Dev Namo" 3 times (Tune on page 143).

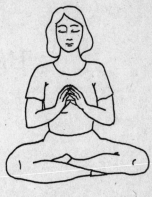

Posture: Sit in Easy Pose or in a chair with your spine straight.

Focus: Look at the tip of your nose.

Breath: Breathe 4 complete breaths per minute in the following way: inhale for 5 seconds, hold for 5 seconds, exhale for 5 seconds. All breathing is done through the nose.

Mantra: This Medical Meditation is done without a mantra.

Mudra: Bring your hands to the center of your chest, with the tips of your thumbs touching each other, and each of your fingertips touching the corresponding finger on your opposite hand. There is a space between your palms, and your fingertips are pointing upward.

Time: 11 minutes.

End: Inhale deeply and hold your breath for 10 seconds, exhale. Repeat 2 more times.

COMMENTS: This Medical Meditation is especially useful for dealing with stressful relationships and with unsettling issues from the past.

CHAPTER FIFTEEN

The Fifth Chakra

The Voice of Truth

A Case History

HEALING WITH THE FIFTH CHAKRA

Harry, a fifty-three-year-old male, had symptoms commonly associated with hypothyroidism. He had begun to gain weight, was somewhat puffy and bloated due to water retention, suffered from constipation due to reduced peristaltic action of the bowel, and was experiencing decreased physical and mental energy. He also had chronic congestion in his throat, and cleared his throat quite frequently.

Harry was treated by a master practitioner of the esoteric method known as Sat Nam Rasayan, an intuitive, distant healing technique. This session centered on healing low ethereal energy in his throat chakra. Harry was also placed on a program of Medical Meditation that focused upon his fifth chakra.

In addition, blood testing was done, which subsequently revealed that Harry's thyroid hormones (T-3 and T-4) were in the low normal range, and that his pituitary's thyroid-stimulating hormone was in the high-normal range (indicating that his pituitary was having to work excessively to stimulate thyroid secretions).

The orthodox medical approach would have been to withhold medication while the patient's hormones were still in the range of normal. However, instead of this approach, which I consider to often be detrimentally conservative, Harry was placed on a very mild program of hormonal replacement therapy.

The integrative approach of Medical Meditation in combination with mild hormone replacement therapy was quite successful. Harry experienced an increase in physical and mental energy and was no longer constipated. His problem with water retention ceased, and he lost his puffy, bloated appearance. His scratchy throat cleared up, and he lost sixteen pounds over approximately the next month, without additional exercise or dieting. His health remains excellent.

The General Characteristics of the Fifth Chakra

One of the most fascinating results of fifth-chakra distress that I have observed clinically is a loss of the so-called twinkle in the eye. It's hard to define exactly what that sparkle in the eye is, because it's a rather amorphous physical condition. It is not simple clarity of the sclera, nor focus of the pupil. Nonetheless, almost anyone can recognize it, and most people are attracted by it.

The loss of the twinkle in the eye is obvious when a person dies. At the moment of death the light in the eyes goes out, and is replaced by a dull glaze that is markedly different from the unfocused stare of a living person.

Since the fifth chakra, or throat chakra, governs the thyroid gland, it would seem possible that the lack of a twinkle in the eye is merely a reflection of low levels of the stimulating thyroid hormones, T-3 and T-4. However, I believe the truth lies deeper. I think that when the throat chakra is dysfunctional, it robs us of the proverbial spark of life that ignites the twinkle in the eye.

The twinkle in the eye, although physically apparent, is essentially an ethereal, nonphysical phenomenon. As such, it is wholly appropriate that it be associated with the fifth chakra, which is more mysterious and magical than any of the chakras below it. The fifth chakra is very much a part of the upper triangle of chakras, which are strongly associated with the mind and spirit. The chakras below the fifth chakra are all ruled by elements that are well within our early, human purview: earth, fire, air, and water. In contrast, the fifth chakra is ruled by the element of ether. Ether, in this context, does not refer to the common gas that has been used as an anesthetic.

Instead, it is the element that the ancient masters considered to be the original substance of the universe (similarly to how modern scientists now consider the void of space to be the original substance of the universe). More precisely, ether was thought to be the condition of time and space that allowed matter to exist.

As you'll recall from the chapter on sound, the original existence of matter was believed by the ancient masters (and a growing legion of quantum physicists) to have sprung from vibration: In the beginning was the Vibration—or the Word.

Thus, according to the cosmology of the masters, the world around us emerged from ether, and was organized by the activity that is most closely associated with the throat chakra: vibration. This world, of course, includes not just the material world but also the ethereal, as evidenced by the root of the word *ethereal:* ether.

By this reckoning, the fifth chakra is closely aligned with the genesis, or seed, of existence. That's one reason why the throat chakra responds so well to the Bij Mantra, or Seed Mantra, "Sat Nam."

This alignment with the ultimate creative force could account for why a strong fifth chakra puts a twinkle in the eye. When the throat chakra is balanced with free-flowing energy, it enables the spark of the human spirit and the spark of the divine spirit to light the fire of life in the eyes. Metaphorically, the creative seed power of the fifth chakra is alluded to in the colloquialism that describes a person's existence before birth: Back when you were just a twinkle in your father's eye.

To be whole and soul, though, the seed of being associated with the throat chakra must be in synchronous vibration with the original Word that organized the matter of the universe: the vibration of divine being. As Dr. Gurucharan has stated, "The power of the fifth chakra is to have your tongue and the tongue of God be the same."

For this to occur, your tongue, and your voice, must speak the truth. This is simply another way of saying that your words must clearly state what is inside you, since your core being is truth. Thus, not only does the fifth chakra empower your ability to speak the truth, but truth empowers the fifth chakra.

Conversely, lies weaken the fifth chakra. All types of false, negative, destructive talk compromise the energy of the throat chakra. When people engage in slander, gossip, and the unfair judging of others, they block fifth-chakra energy, and prevent ethereal energy from rising past the fifth chakra to the highest energy centers. This impedes spiritual growth, and it also causes physical harm to the system. As a rule, this harm is most keenly felt in the major physical structures of the throat chakra: the thyroid gland, the parathyroid gland, the trachea and larynx, and the cervical vertebrae. However, because all the chakras work in harmony, a blockage in any of them, including the fifth chakra, can cause problems elsewhere.

One form of lie that is particularly harmful is a negative, self-destructive statement about oneself. Unfortunately, though, many people tend to frequently indulge in this negative self-talk. They tell themselves crippling lies, such as: "I could never do that," or "I always make this mistake, and probably always will." These self-fulfilling prophecies not only undercut the power of the psyche, but also weaken the ethereal energy of the fifth-chakra organs that utter them.

If you find yourself frequently engaging in negative self-talk, you should make a strong effort to reverse it. Tell yourself, "I can do this," or "Success comes easily to me. I don't have to struggle." These simple affirmations will not only reprogram your psyche for success but bring power to your throat chakra. It's easy, of course, to be cynical, and to try to protect your feelings with pessimism. But pessimism is ultimately a lie. Life is good. It's that simple—and people who let themselves pollute this simple truth with pessimistic fear are just hiding from reality.

If you simply can't make yourself abandon negative self-talk, try to stop talking altogether for an entire day. This alone will restore some power to your throat chakra, and is an excellent exercise for learning that the only proper use of the throat chakra is to express truth.

Another extremely common type of lie is the prideful statement, which is usually a defensive posture intended to hide insecurity. As a rule, the most outwardly prideful people are the most inwardly full of doubt. Even if these arrogant people really do have a lot to be proud of—money, power, fame—these trappings of success are often just the hard-won cloaks that they were desperate to accumulate to cover their inner emptiness.

Pride is a rope of many strands, and the ancient masters identified the nine most common strands of pride: (1) in physique and strength; (2) in intellect; (3) in morals and virtues; (4) in psychic power; (5) in spirituality; (6) in social status; (7) in wealth and possessions; and (8) in beauty or handsomeness.

These conditions of being are all wonderful attributes, and are not to be slighted or ignored. But they should not be mentioned with pride. They should be mentioned with gratitude. Pride is a lie. Gratitude is truth.

The Bible says, Pride goeth before a fall. This figurative truth may also apply quite literally to the chakra system. When pride blocks the upward flow of healing kundalini energy, this energy must necessarily fall back to the lower chakras, where it will remain, trapped and stagnant as mind, body, and spirit wither.

Pride, as well as other manifestations of egotism, also interferes with the ability to properly hear, which is another vital function governed by the fifth chakra. Frequently, people with imbalance in the fifth chakra find it very hard to listen to others, much preferring to have others listen to them.

Again, the most important physical structure governed by the fifth chakra is the thyroid, which controls the metabolic rate. If the thyroid is overactive, it can result in the condition of hyperthyroidism, which is characterized by an accelerated metabolism, weight loss, hyperactivity, and agitation. If the thyroid is underactive (a far more common condition), it can result in hypothyroidism, which is characterized by a slow metabolism, weight gain, sluggishness, and depression.

Thyroid function, and therefore metabolic rate, are affected by the ethereal energies of the throat chakra. If the throat chakra is weak in ethereal energy, it can weaken the thyroid. This can contribute to the common condition of hypothyroidism. If the throat chakra is overactive, it can contribute to the opposite condition of hyperthyroidism.

Just as the throat chakra is associated with the physical aspects of metabolism, it is also associated with the ethereal metabolism—the metabolic rate of the ethereal body. The throat chakra is a nexus for upward-bound energies arriving from the lower chakras, and downward-bound energies arriving from the upper chakras. In the vortex of the throat chakra, these energies are swirled and mixed, broken down, and put back together. Then they are expressed, via one's voice, as the special, original, signature sound of each person. This is an essentially metabolic function, similar in action to the physical metabolism governed by the thyroid. Thus, in the metabolic process of refining one's ethereal energies, a person also defines his or her personality.

This self-defining process is dependent upon many factors, but one that is especially important is the human will. Despite the power of fate, we are all ultimately what we will ourselves to be. Therefore, the throat chakra is also often perceived as the primary site of the will. After all, a great deal of willpower is needed to honestly and outwardly express the truth that lies within. While this truth is still inside, we are safe from backlash and criticism. But when we assert ourselves, and express our innermost feelings, we become vulnerable.

This vulnerability points once again to the importance of truthfulness. If our self-expression is based on truth, we will be ultimately aligned with the power of the universe, even if we do face worldly attack from our detractors. But if our self-expression is a lie, we will be ultimately aligned against the power of the universe. Only the truth survives. Only the truth endures.

The Physical Characteristics of the Fifth Chakra

The most important physical structures governed by the fifth chakra, in terms of whole-body systemic function, are the thyroid and parathyroid glands. The thyroid is especially important, since it establishes the basic metabolic rate.

The thyroid produces thyroid hormones, which control the relative speed of the metabolism and also help control body temperature. In addition, the thyroid hormones raise the level of enzymes in every cell's energy-producing mitochondria. This increases oxygen utilization in the cells, and stimulates energy and metabolism.

The incidence of poor thyroid function in modern society appears to be quite high. Some researchers have estimated that up to 40 percent of the population suffers from at least mild dysfunction of the thyroid, and they believe this problem is part of the reason so many people are overweight. This estimate is considered too high by most orthodox physicians, but many doctors of integrative medicine agree that low-grade thyroid dysfunction is relatively common. One reason for poor thyroid function is insufficient intake of the minerals zinc and selenium. Another is reduced blood flow to the thyroid. Medical Meditation, however, is probably the best single physical therapy for restoring blood flow to the thyroid (and parathyroid), because kundalini yoga exercises are virtually the only exercises ever designed specifically to increase the flow of blood (as well as ethereal energy) to the various components of the endocrine system, including the thyroid.

When ethereal energy to the throat chakra is deficient, it can result in insufficient thyroid function (or hypothyroidism). It can also result in degenerative diseases of all the other glands and organs governed by the throat chakra. Conversely, when ethereal energy becomes trapped in the throat chakra, and builds to excessive levels, it can result in hyperthyroidism, or overactivity of the thyroid, which is characterized by agitation and hyperactivity. Excessive ethereal energy can also contribute to inflammatory conditions, including thyroiditis.

The parathyroid has a less pronounced systemic effect, but is still vitally important. Its primary function is to govern calcium metabolism, which also indirectly affects the metabolism of magnesium. Parathyroid hormone, or PTH, controls calcium metabolism in bone and muscle cells. Although this may seem to be a rather limited function, it's really quite important. When the parathyroid glands were removed from animals in laboratory experiments, the animals quickly began to suffer from lethargy, anorexia, vomiting, temperature drop, and muscle spasms. Within a few days, they suffered cardiac failure and paralysis of the respiratory muscles, and died.

Even a mild deficit of PTH can cause bone loss, which contributes to onset of osteoporosis and can cause cramping in muscles. Muscle cramping, particularly of the legs, is quite common among older people, due in part to atrophy of the parathyroid during the aging process. This glandular decline interferes with calcium metabolism and may produce the condition of hypocalcemic tetany. It is my clinical opinion that this atrophy due to aging can be significantly ameliorated with Medical Meditation.

Other diseases of the fifth-chakra structures include chronic laryngitis, parathyroid gland lesions, esophageal cancer, and laryngeal cancer.

The final important physical problem that can be caused by energy imbalance in the throat chakra is interference with the tenth cranial nerve, or vagus nerve, which travels through the jaw area on its way to the most important organs of the chest and abdomen, including the heart, lungs, and stomach. Proper function of the vagus nerve is extremely important for optimal function of these vital abdominal organs. In addition, the vagus nerve is responsible for much of the parasympathetic branch innervation of the internal organs. This parasympathetic innervation is critically important to good health, since the parasympathetic branch is the primary governor of the body's healing, rest-and-repair mechanisms.

Following are Medical Meditations and kundalini yoga exercises that are especially appropriate for the fifth chakra.

Medical Meditations for the Fifth Chakra

SPECIAL MEDITATION FOR THE FIFTH CHAKRA

Tune in and center yourself by chanting "Ong Namo, Guru Dev Namo" 3 times (Tune on page 143).

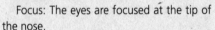

Posture: Sit in Easy Pose or in a chair with a straight spine. Your neck is absolutely straight, with your chin pulled in; this is the neck lock. Your chin rests in the notch of your collarbone. Your head stays level without tilting forward. Your spine in the neck is straight. Your chin is pulled in, your chest is out, and there is little weight on the buttocks. When the neck lock is properly applied, a stretch can be felt in your deltoid muscles.

Focus: The eyes are focused at the tip of the nose.

Breath: The breath will come automatically as you chant.

Mantra: "Hummee Hum, Brahm Hum." This is chanted with the root of your tongue, and the pressure is felt in your throat.

Meaning of mantra: "We are we, and we are one." On a higher spiritual level, it means, we are already everything we need to be.

Mudra: Hands are relaxed on the knees in gyan mudra, with the index fingers touching the thumbs.

Time: 11 minutes.

End: Inhale, hold your breath for 10 seconds, exhale. Meditate silently for a few minutes.

COMMENTS: Practicing this Medical Meditation for 11 minutes a day, for 18 months, will keep you young in spirit, with a youthful look.

> Those who do not know how to live up to their words shall never have the knowledge of God.
> —*Yogi Bhajan*

TWO MEDICAL MEDITATIONS TO OPEN THE HIGHER CENTERS

Tune in and center yourself by chanting "Ong Namo, Guru Dev Namo" 3 times (Tune on page 143).

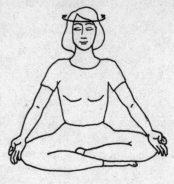

1. Posture: Sit in Easy Pose or in a chair with your spine straight.

Focus: The eyes are closed and focused at the third-eye point.

Breath: The breath will come automatically as you chant.

Mantra: Begin with your head facing forward. Then turn it to the right shoulder 4 times and chant "Sat Nam" each time. Next, turn to the left 4 times and chant "Wahe Guru" each time. The mantra will be a rhythmic "Sat Nam, Sat Nam, Sat Nam, Sat Nam, Wahe Guru, Wahe Guru, Wahe Guru, Wahe Guru."

Meaning of mantra: "My true identity brings me from darkness to the light."

Mudra: Your hands are resting on your knees in gyan mudra, with your index fingers touching your thumbs. Your arms are straight.

Time: Continue in a regular rhythm for 6 minutes.

End: Inhale to the center, hold your breath for 10 seconds, exhale.

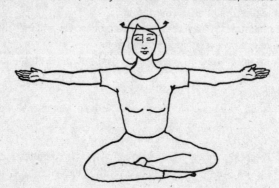

2. Posture: Sit in Easy Pose or in a chair with your spine straight. Extend your arms to your sides, parallel to the ground.

Focus: Concentrate on the top center of your head, and at the same time be aware of the energy in your palms.

Breath: The breath will come automatically as you chant.

Mantra: Do the same head movement as above, but use the mantra "Whaho" every time you turn left, and "Guru" when you turn right. This time it will be a continuous "Whaho, Whaho, Whaho, Whaho, Guru, Guru, Guru, Guru."

Meaning of mantra: "Hail the infinite wisdom."

Mudra: The palms are flat and face up.

Time: 6 minutes.

End: Inhale deeply and relax your breath and arms. Continue to meditate within the self for a few minutes.

COMMENTS: When the thyroid and parathyroid secretions are stimulated to a certain level, the pranic energy flows more freely into the upper energy centers of the heart. The first meditation has this effect. The second meditation focuses on the heart center energy of compassion, and the healing energy of the hands. Both meditations increase the circulation of blood to the brain. They are excellent as short meditations in themselves, or as a preparation for a longer meditation. Both Medical Meditations clear the mind and allow greater concentration.

MEDICAL MEDITATION FOR
GLANDULAR BALANCE AND BLISS

Tune in and center yourself by chanting "Ong Namo, Guru Dev Namo" 3 times (Tune on page 143).

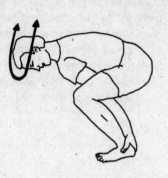

1. Posture: From a standing position, go into Chair Pose: knees bent, back parallel to the ground, hands grasping your heels firmly. Keep your spine straight, and lock your head down. Turn your head to the left shoulder and say "Wahe," turn your head to the right shoulder and say "Guru."

Focus: The eyes are closed and focused at the third-eye point.

Breath: The breath will come automatically as you chant.

Mantra: "Wahe Guru."

Meaning of mantra: "Ecstasy of infinite consciousness."

Mudra: The hands are clasping your heels.

Time: 1–3 minutes.

End: Inhale to the center, hold your breath for 10 seconds, exhale.

Continue the head movement to maintain a continuous sound current—"Wahe Guru, Wahe Guru, Wahe Guru." If you cannot do this position, you can sit in a chair.

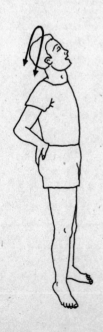

2. Posture: Stand up straight and lean backward. Keep your legs straight and let your head fall back.

Focus: The eyes are closed and focused at the third-eye point.

Breath: The breath will come automatically as you chant.

Mantra: "Wahe Guru." Coordinate the same head movement and mantra as above.

Mudra: Place your hands on your lower back for support.

Time: 1–3 minutes.

End: Inhale to the center, hold your breath for 10 seconds, exhale.

3. Posture: From a standing position, bend forward until your hands touch your knees. Keep your back straight, but bend your head up.

Focus: The eyes are closed and focused at the third-eye point.

Breath: The breath will come automatically as you chant.

Mantra: "Wahe Guru." Coordinate the same head movement and mantra as above.

Mudra: Rest your hands on your knees for support.

Time: 1–3 minutes.

End: Inhale to the center, hold your breath for 10 seconds, exhale.

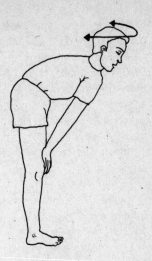

4. Posture: Stand up and stretch your arms overhead as to touch the sky. Chant "Wahe" and keep your feet flat on the floor, chant "Guru" and rise up on your toes.

Focus: The eyes are closed and focused at the third-eye point.

Breath: The breath will come automatically as you chant.

Mantra: "Wahe Guru."

Mudra: The hands and fingers are stretched up.

Time: 1–3 minutes.

End: Inhale in the starting position, hold your breath for 10 seconds, and stretch your arms up, exhale, and relax.

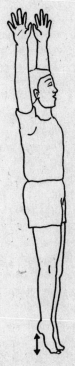

5. Posture: Sit on your heels and place your palms flat on the floor just in front of your knees. Keep your spine and your arms straight. On this up position, chant "Wahe." Then bend forward to touch your forehead to the ground and chant "Guru."

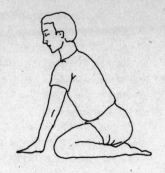

Focus: The eyes are closed and focused at the third-eye point.

Breath: The breath will come automatically as you chant.

Mantra: "Wahe Guru."

Mudra: The hands are flat on the floor in front of you.

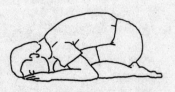

Time: 1–3 minutes.

End: Inhale, hold your breath for 10 seconds, exhale.

If you cannot sit in this position, you may do this exercise sitting in a chair. In this case, place your hands on your knees and bend forward as much as possible.

6. Posture: Sit in Easy Pose or in a chair with your spine straight.

Focus: The eyes are closed and focused at the third-eye point.

Breath: The breath will come automatically as you chant.

Mantra: "Sa Ta Na Ma."

Meaning of mantra: This mantra represents the cycle of creation: *Sa* means infinity; *Ta* means life; *Na* means death; *Ma* means rebirth.

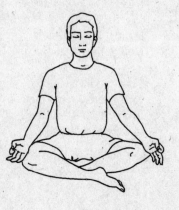

Mudra: Your hands are relaxed on your knees in gyan mudra, with your index fingers touching your thumbs.

Time: Whisper the mantra for 2 minutes, then chant it loudly for 2 minutes more.

End: Inhale, hold your breath for 10 seconds, exhale.

7. Posture: Immediately sit on your heels, keeping your spine straight. Flex your spine forward and whisper "Sa," flex backward and whisper "Ta," then forward and whisper "Na," finally backward and whisper "Ma."

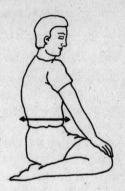

Focus: The eyes are closed and focused at the third-eye point.

Breath: The breath will come automatically as you chant.

Mantra: "Sa Ta Na Ma" is chanted with a powerful whisper.

Mudra: Place your hands flat on your thighs.

Time: 1–3 minutes.

End: Inhale in the starting position, hold your breath for 10 seconds, exhale, and relax.

COMMENTS: This Medical Meditation is known only by experiencing it. Basically, the set is a total workout for the thyroid, the pituitary, and the pineal glands. Your whole body will sweat. Meditation after this kriya brings the realization that we are channels for truth, and that to maintain grace in the most ungraceful moments is the true human worth.

This is a very physical meditation. If you have any neck or back problems, or injuries, be very careful. Proceed very slowly and reduce the time of each exercise. This blissful meditation is also appropriate for the seventh and eighth chakras.

MEDICAL MEDITATION FOR THE THYROID GLAND

Tune in and center yourself by chanting "Ong Namo, Guru Dev Namo" 3 times (Tune on page 143).

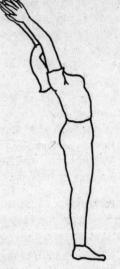

1. Posture: Stand up and extend your arms up and back, arching back 20 degrees from your standing position. Your head is aligned with the body. Hold the position.

Focus: The eyes are closed and focused at the third-eye point, or slightly open for balance, if necessary.

Breath: Long, slow, deep breathing through the nose.

Mantra: This Medical Meditation is done without a mantra.

Mudra: Same as posture.

Time: 1–2 minutes.

End: Inhale deeply, hold your breath for 5 seconds, exhale, and move immediately into the next position.

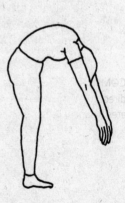

2. Posture: Still standing up, very, very slowly bend forward to your maximum extent, keeping your arms straight and close to the ears.

Focus: The eyes are closed and focused at the third-eye point, or slightly open for balance, if necessary.

Breath: All breathing is done through the nose. Inhale deeply, hold the breath and pump the navel as long as possible. Exhale, hold your breath out, and pump the navel again. Continue this cycle.

Mantra: This Medical Meditation is done without a mantra.

Mudra: Same as posture.

Time: 1–2 minutes.

End: Inhale, hold your breath for 5 seconds, exhale and relax.

COMMENTS : Along with the parathyroid gland, the thyroid gland is the guardian of health and beauty. Improper balance of these two glands can make you age before your time. The skin, the complexion, and the outward appearance are affected by the thyroid. This Medical Meditation is also called Miracle Bend; its other benefits are to promote emotional and mental balance, as well as prevention of early menopause.

MEDICAL MEDITATION FOR THE PARATHYROID GLAND

Tune in and center yourself by chanting "Ong Namo, Guru Dev Namo" 3 times (Tune on page 143).

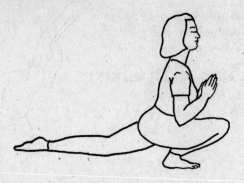

Posture: Crouch down on your right leg, with your left leg extended back, trailing behind you like a tail. Your left knee is off the floor.

Focus: Focus at the tip of the nose.

Breath: Long, slow, and deep breathing through the nose.

Mantra: As you inhale, mentally say "Ra," as you exhale, mentally say "Ma."

Meaning of mantra: "The energy of the totality of the sun and moon."

Mudra: The hands are in Prayer Pose at the chest, palms touching.

Time: 3–11 minutes.

End: Inhale deeply, hold your breath for 10 seconds, exhale, and relax.

COMMENTS: This Medical Meditation is known as Siam Kriya; it was taught to direct the flow of healing energy to the side where it is primarily needed. This creates balance, rather than repeating it on the other side.

CHAPTER SIXTEEN

The Sixth Chakra

The Path of the Soul

A Case History

HEALING WITH THE SIXTH CHAKRA

Janet, a middle-aged woman, first began to experience symptoms of pain, muscle spasm, and fatigue in 1987. Unable to perform even her simplest household chores, she consulted a variety of doctors. One prescribed muscle relaxants, which did not help. Another recommended exercises, visualization, and biofeedback, but none of these worked. In fact, the neck exercises that were prescribed made the pain in her neck so severe that she was unable to turn it from side to side. An orthopedic specialist suggested hydrotherapy, but it too seemed to exacerbate the pain. A psychiatrist prescribed analgesic drugs, but, as Janet later recalled, "I refused to live on pills for the rest of my life. I never filled the prescription."

Her pain and stiffness limited her life terribly. She could not sit in a chair for more than ten minutes, and was unable to ride in a car for more than twenty minutes.

She later recalled, "It was a terrible time. I was told not to lift more than five pounds. To get out of bed in the morning, I needed my husband to lift me by my head and back. Several times during the night also, he had to do this, to help me change my position. I remember hurting so much that his hands on me felt like daggers. The spasms were so bad that one night we called for an ambulance, but they couldn't move me to take me to the hospital. Still, I was afraid to take drugs for the pain, because I was afraid of becoming addicted."

Finally, Janet consulted another doctor, a neurologist, who correctly diagnosed her problem as fibromyalgia, a condition that causes widespread muscle pain. Approximately 20 percent of all fibromyalgia patients are disabled by the disorder. It strikes mostly women, and is now believed to often be associated with low levels of the neurotransmitter serotonin.

At this time, Janet sought consultation for Medical Meditation. She still remembers her first meditation clearly: "It was an experience I'll never forget. It felt as if someone had lifted me off the floor, and I was floating in a circle of light. I saw God in a white gown, hovering over me. It was so intense, as if He were saying, 'You're OK now; you're in the right place.' I thought I'd died and gone to heaven—all white light around me! When the meditation was over, I didn't want to move. That was six years ago, and my life changed forever. I got home that night, and it was like my body was light."

She soon overcame the severe, crippling aspects of her pain. She began to function normally.

The only noticeable sign of her fibromyalgia is occasional, moderate stiffness in her neck and shoulders. However, as she states, "I can get rid of it. The breathing is so important, and so is the meditation. I am in control of me, my body, and my mind. I am able to do all my own housework, but I've learned to seek a balance in everything I do. I get the right amount of rest, and I walk. Meditation is so enlightening!"

Janet actually healed the dysfunctional mechanisms in her body that were creating the pain. This probably involved increasing her levels of the neurotransmitter serotonin. Serotonin is now well known to many people as a contentment chemical, mostly because of the popularity of drugs such as Prozac, which boost serotonin levels. However, serotonin also has a number of important physical effects throughout the body. For example, it regulates blood vessel elasticity, which helps prevent migraines. It also indirectly helps repair minor muscle tears, which prevents ongoing fibromyalgia. Therefore, increasing serotonin by bringing energy to the sixth chakra has far-reaching effects, in every part of the body. This is one reason the sixth chakra is so important: it can help the whole body to heal.

Over time, Janet gained the ability to activate her sixth chakra so fully that she became virtually impervious to even the most severe pain. Her abilities were put to the test, though, when she went to her dentist for root canal surgery—and requested that he use no anesthetic.

The dentist refused to do so. After all, in a root canal procedure, the tooth is drilled all the way to the pulp, where a highly sensitive nerve is situated. Direct contact with the nerve is invariably excruciating, unless the nerve is completely deadened with novocaine. Furthermore, most patients also require an additional analgesic, nitrous oxide, to help their brains reinterpret the stress signals that emanate from the distressed nerve.

Janet, however, would not consent to any anesthesia. She convinced her doctor to at least begin the surgery without anesthetic, and promised that she would request novocaine if it became painful. The dentist reluctantly agreed.

Janet asked the dentist to leave the room for twenty minutes, and to then begin the surgery without speaking or interrupting her thoughts.

When the dentist left the room, Janet began to concentrate on her sixth chakra, located in the area behind her forehead, while she focused on a specific image: "I put myself in another place, my garden, where there are beautiful flowers of all colors, and where I lay in a long, white silk dress as a breeze flowed over me, just to cool me from the warm sun. White clouds floated through the blue sky, and water gently flicked at my toes."

The dentist entered the room, and began to drill.

By the time Janet emerged from her meditation, the procedure was complete. She had experienced absolutely no pain.

The dentist was astonished, and agreed to do further dental work on her without anesthetic. This work included deep fillings, and even crowns. Each time, the dentist's colleagues were called into the room to witness this incredible feat. Janet later remarked, "The other dentists were amazed, and tried to understand. I just told them, it's the power of the mind."

The General Characteristics of the Sixth Chakra

The power of the mind! Nothing on the earthly plane is more extraordinary! The mind is the ultimate repository of human consciousness and the human spirit. This consciousness and spirit encompass our capacity for cognition, emotion, will, and even contact with the ethereal.

Thus, it is little wonder that the sixth chakra, or *ajna*, which encompasses the brain, is the focal point for some of our most highly developed ethereal energy. Only the crown chakra and the aura, which are in communion with the divine spirit, hold higher energies.

The sixth chakra is commonly referred to as the third-eye chakra, because of its link to the quality of intuition. It governs the pituitary gland, the master gland of the endocrine system. The pituitary is also associated with intuition, partly because it, more than any other single physical structure, is the link between mind and body. The pituitary translates the ideas and emotions of the brain's cortex into the chemicals that control mood, muscle, and metabolism.

The ancient masters did not know about the pituitary, but they did believe that very special fluids issued forth from the sixth chakra. They called these fluids the *amrit,* meaning ambrosia, or nectar. We now know that this nectar consists of pituitary secretions that enter the bloodstream and travel throughout the body, directing the actions of all the other endocrine glands.

The pituitary's secretions are among the most important of the molecules of emotion, and molecules of knowledge. Pituitary secretions literally inform the body's other glands and organs about what the brain wants the body to do. These other glands and organs, in turn, have a fundamental thinking capability all their own (mediated by neuropeptides, neurotransmitters, and neurohormones). This nonbrain thinking that occurs throughout the body almost certainly plays a role in intuition. For example, your intestinal neuropeptides probably contribute to your proverbial gut feelings.

The intuition that can be reached through the sixth chakra is, however, widely misunderstood. Most people think intuition applies primarily to mysterious extrasensory abilities, such as precognition, the ability to know something before it happens. This is part of what intuition is, but it's not the most important part.

The most significant aspect of intuition is the ability to see from the soul instead of the ego. When your abiding perspective is from your soul, you make decisions, naturally and effortlessly, that favor your soul over your ego. You focus on the entirety of your being, rather than on your narrow, ego-based concerns about survival and status. Then, if you are strong, and have a firm foundation of lower-triangle chakras, you act on these decisions. I call this Taking the Path of the Soul.

When you take the path of the soul, you eventually decrease the distance between your ego and your inner divinity, or cosmic spark. As this distance decreases, you become aware of the cosmic spark that exists in every other person and every other entity in the universe. This creates a merging of all things. I refer to this merging as truth.

Many people don't share this definition of truth. They believe that truth consists simply of honest expression. But there is far more to truth than just telling the truth. Real truth means living the truth. To live the truth, you must recognize your own divine essence, and the divine essence of all others. This alone will enable you to experience the reality of oneness.

When you do experience oneness, or the merging of all things, you will achieve ultimate human consciousness. This consciousness naturally leads to dignity, or power over one's material desires. Dignity can then lead to divinity. And divinity gives you the strength and compassion to sacrifice, which ultimately engenders service to others, happiness, and optimal health.

As consciousness begins to unfold, it opens the intuitive mind—the complete mind—and reveals a vast panorama of reality that had once been hidden. Quite simply, with full consciousness, we see more. We see beyond the obvious. We see the textures and nuances that often escape notice by the brain's frontal cortex, which is able to recognize only what it's been taught to recognize through prior experience.

With this new vision of reality, we can make new choices, including the choices that line the path of the soul. With this panoply of new choices, we can in effect create our own new reality. This was what happened to the patient who underwent root canal surgery without anesthetic. She transcended the mundane reality of her pain and suffering, and emerged in a higher reality of peace and joy.

In certain trendy, soft-minded New Age circles, the phrase "create your own reality" is bandied about so haphazardly that it means almost nothing. To some people, it consists of little more than wishful thinking: "If I just think I'm rich, it'll happen!" These people are missing the point. The true essence of creating your own reality means responding to the real world with your highest self, which will elevate you to the best part of that world—the healthy, happy, holy part. This part of your world already exists. It's within you now, awaiting your arrival. But there is only one path to it: the path of the soul. The sixth chakra is the doorway that opens onto that path. When the sixth chakra is balanced, the door opens.

When you open and balance the sixth chakra, and walk the path of the soul, you attain freedom from all worldly limitations, including those that limit healing, happiness, prosperity, and wisdom. You create inner harmony and peace of mind.

The mental energy that is created by Medical Meditation can open the sixth chakra. This energy is very powerful, very focused, and more useful than a laser. When the sixth chakra is open, the physical body—including the brain—becomes a tool for what we can truly call, by now, the spiritual life.

On a practical level, after all your lower chakras are open, and your sixth chakra opens, you can maximize your inner power to heal. After all, *all* healing begins in the mind. And the mind begins in the sixth chakra.

The Physical Characteristics of the Sixth Chakra

Because all healing begins in the mind, the energy of the sixth chakra can heal not only physical structures that are located within the sixth chakra but also dysfunction throughout the body.

To do this, though, the pituitary must be functioning optimally, since it is the single most important link between mind and body. The pituitary is vitally connected to the section of your brain known as the limbic system. While the neocortex of the brain is essentially your thinking brain, the limbic system is your feeling brain. The limbic system controls not only emotions but also memory. It houses the hippocampus, where short-term memories are shipped to long-term storage in the neocortex.

The limbic system is one of the brain's three basic components. The other two are the thinking neocortex and the reptilian brain stem. In evolution, the first to exist was the brain stem, which arose in reptiles and governs primitive, survival-oriented actions. Reptiles are utterly without emotion. The second part of the brain that evolved was the limbic system, which endows warm-blooded animals with the capacity for emotion. The last part of the brain to evolve was the neocortex, which gave rise to advanced logic in humans.

The limbic system, influenced by the pituitary, is so important that it is sometimes called the second brain. The interlinked system of brain structures that compose the limbic system literally has a mind of its own. This mind has the physical capacity to transfer its knowledge to the rest of the body, via the endocrine system.

The endocrine system is the network of glands that secretes hormones directly into the bloodstream. These hormones are signaling chemicals that activate organs throughout the body. Among the most important endocrine glands are the adrenals, which trigger the fight-or-flight response; the thymus, which coordinates the immune response; the thyroid, which governs metabolism; the gonads, which orchestrate sexual function; and the pineal, which helps regulate sleep.

Besides affecting the body, hormones also act directly upon the brain. For example, high estrogen levels contribute to increased verbal dexterity. Similarly, adequate levels of testosterone contribute to the emotional experience of well-being, in both males and females.

Controlling all of these endocrine glands, though, is the pituitary in the sixth chakra. The pituitary, which is approximately the size of a pea, is located near the middle of the brain, with the other limbic structures. The pituitary secretes a number of hormones, some of which act directly upon organs, and some of which activate other endocrine glands.

The pituitary is directed by the brain through the hypothalamus, which influences pituitary secretions. The primary effects of the pituitary, though, occur throughout the body. Therefore, the pituitary is an integral part of both mind and body.

If the ethereal energy in the sixth chakra is imbalanced, or low, it can harm the function of the pituitary. When this happens, the mind-body link is severely compromised. In effect, the body doesn't know what the mind is thinking, and the mind doesn't know what the body is doing. When the mind-body link is disturbed, one's capacity for intuition is badly hampered. The mind and body no longer function as a single, synchronous unit, and this robs the brain of the feedback from the body that it needs to make wise, intuitive decisions.

On a purely physical level, disturbance of the pituitary can trigger a wide range of endocrinologic disorders. This can result in metabolic problems such as hypothyroidism or hyperthyroidism. It can also result in agitation, anxiety, depression, impaired libido, insomnia, and a number of other problems that are triggered by endocrine imbalance.

Dysfunction of the sixth chakra can also result in memory dysfunction. My extensive work with Alzheimer's patients, as well as patients in various stages of the ubiquitous condition of age-associated memory disorder, has led me to believe that sixth-chakra dysfunction is a major element in memory loss. In innumerable cases, my patients with memory loss have benefited tremendously from Medical Meditations that focus primarily upon the sixth chakra, and in particular from the vibratory effects of chanting. As I've mentioned, the pituitary is in very close physical proximity to the nasal and throat cavities, and to the bony structures of the skull, all of which are strongly impacted by vibratory chanting. These vibrations imbue the pituitary with notably increased blood flow, and also bring ethereal energy surging into the sixth chakra.

Increased blood flow to the head also helps to strengthen and tone the arteries that supply blood to the brain. This not only increases cognitive energy but may also help prevent strokes. Kundalini yoga exercises, which are used in Medical Meditation, are virtually the only form of exercise that focus specifically on increasing blood flow to the head.

Another significant side benefit of increased blood flow to the head is the prevention of migraine headaches. Migraines, essentially a disorder of impaired cerebral blood flow, occur when the blood vessels to the brain contract and then suddenly expand to compensate for this contraction. The sudden expansion presses against nerves, and causes severe pain.

Besides improving cognition, or thinking, sixth-chakra Medical Meditations also improve other neurological functions. Medical Meditation is especially adept at ameliorating emotional disorders, including clinical depression and anxiety. Unlike virtually any other modality, it simultaneously addresses both the physical and mental components of emotional disorders. It helps patients to rebalance their brain chemistries at the same time that it helps them recognize and change the psychological and behavioral elements of their disorders.

Medical Meditation can also help improve the clinical profile of strictly physical neurological disorders, such as multiple sclerosis. Used as an adjunctive therapy, Medical Meditation has helped some MS patients to retard the progression of the disease, and to mute its symptoms.

For many years, I have also treated a wide variety of other chronic pain disorders with Medical Meditation. As I wrote in *The Pain Cure,* pain is in the brain. To some extent, almost all chronic pain is at least the partial result of a failure of the pain-blocking mechanisms of the brain. In chronic pain patients, the biological gates of pain, which normally block pain from the brain, are overwhelmed. However, Medical Meditation helps to strengthen the gates of pain, and can thus be extremely helpful for a wide variety of other forms of pain. For about seven years, during the late 1980s and early 1990s, when my practice focused primarily upon the treatment of patients with chronic pain, I prescribed Medical Meditation to almost all of my pain patients. In a remarkable number of cases, this approach achieved extraordinary medical outcomes.

Thus, as you can see, Medical Meditations that focus on the sixth chakra have a markedly wide-ranging effect. They are not only effective against discrete maladies of the brain—such as memory problems, emotional disorders, endocrine disturbances, and headaches—but also have a powerful impact upon the entire body, since body and mind are one.

Medical Meditations for the Sixth Chakra

SPECIAL MEDITATION FOR THE SIXTH CHAKRA

Tune in and center yourself by chanting "Ong Namo, Guru Dev Namo" 3 times (Tune on page 143).

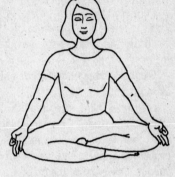

Posture: Sit in Easy Pose or in a chair with your spine straight.

Focus: Look at the tip of your nose (the lotus tip).

Breath: Long, slow, and deep breathing through the nose.

Mantra: This Medical Meditation is done without a mantra.

Mudra: The hands are relaxed on your knees in gyan mudra, with your index fingers touching your thumbs.

Time: 11 minutes.

End: Inhale, hold your breath for 10 seconds, exhale, and relax.

COMMENTS: It is said that by practicing this Medical Meditation between the hours of 4:00 A.M. and 6:00 A.M. local time, you will control the entire glandular system for the next twenty-four hours. This means that glandular secretions will be released in exactly the right amounts. As this occurs, the chemistry of your blood will change for the better.

MEDICAL MEDITATION TO INCREASE COGNITIVE FUNCTION

Tune in and center yourself by chanting "Ong Namo, Guru Dev Namo" 3 times (Tune on page 143).

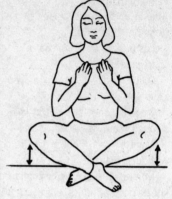

Posture: Sit in Easy Pose or in a chair with your spine straight. Each time you touch your fingers you should also move your knees up and down, like a butterfly flapping its wings. If you are sitting in a chair, smoothly bring your knees together and apart with the chanting.

Focus: The eyes are focused at the tip of the nose.

Breath: The breath will come automatically as you chant.

Mantra: Chant the mantra "Hummee Hum, Brahm Hum." Chant touching the tip of your tongue to your upper palate. When properly chanted in this manner, it will sound strange. One word of the mantra corresponds to one touch of finger and thumb.

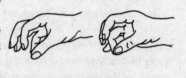

Meaning of mantra: "We are we, and we are one." On a higher spiritual level, it means we are already everything we need to be.

Mudra: Bring your hands to your neck level in front of you, palms facing yourself. Each time you sing a syllable, you touch your fingers in sequence to your thumb, but you skip the ring finger. First touch your thumb and little finger (Mercury finger), then touch your thumb and middle finger (Saturn finger), and then touch your thumb and the index finger (Jupiter finger). Continue the sequence, but do not touch your thumb and ring finger (Sun finger).

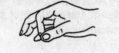

Time: 11 minutes.

End: Inhale, hold your breath for 10 seconds, exhale, and relax.

COMMENTS: This Medical Meditation will increase the hemispheric balance of the brain, and increase attention span. This is a very good exercise for someone suffering from age-associated memory loss, mild cognitive impairment, or early-stage Alzheimer's disease.

MEDICAL MEDITATION TO BALANCE AND RECHARGE
THE NERVOUS AND IMMUNE SYSTEMS

Tune in and center yourself by chanting "Ong Namo, Guru Dev Namo" 3 times
(Tune on page 143).

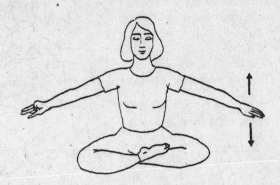

1. Posture: Sit in Easy Pose or in a chair. Place the arms out straight, parallel to the
floor, at 30 degrees from the sides, in a line with the thighs.

Focus: The eyes are closed and focused at the third-eye point.

Breath: Breathe rapidly in sync with the movement of the left arm—it will
become like Breath of Fire, with the navel automatically jumping. The breath
should be loud and strong, almost like a steam engine.

Mantra: This Medical Meditation is done without a mantra.

Mudra: Right hand: palm facing forward, keep index and middle finger stiff and
straight, bending the ring and little fingers into the palm, held by your thumb.
Your arm and the extended fingers remain straight and rigid, and do not move
through the meditation. (Imagine you are shooting a derringer.) Left hand: keep
your elbow straight with palm facing the floor. Move your left arm rapidly up and
down, about 9 inches total.

Time: 11 minutes.

End: Inhale, solidify the body, and, keeping the attention at the third-eye point,
tense every muscle to rebuild the body. Hold 30 seconds and exhale. Immediately
inhale and hold 20 seconds. The last time, rapidly exhale, inhale and hold 5 seconds, exhale, and relax.

2. Posture: Sit in Easy Pose or in a chair with your spine straight.

Focus: The eyes are closed and focused at the third-eye point.

Breath: Inhale through the nose and press the hands together so hard that the
hands, arms, and rib cage begin to shake. Hold 15 seconds and relax.

Mantra: This Medical Meditation is done without a mantra.

Mudra: Lock palm over palm, with right palm facing body, fingers overlapping the back of the opposite hand at the heart center.

Time: Repeat 3 times.

End: Inhale, hold your breath for 10 seconds without pressing the hands together, exhale, and relax.

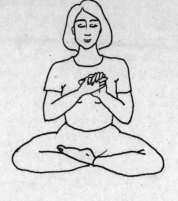

COMMENTS: This is a very precious Medical Meditation. It balances the three activating powers, the three nervous systems of the body; parasympathetic, sympathetic, and voluntary. These are very important and must be in balance.

Do this Medical Meditation so you will never be in pain. It will slowly and steadily build very strong, steel-like stamina in you. You'll think better, act better, and be more intuitive. This exercise is for the spine, which controls the nervous system. It will help balance every cell in your body.

Part 1: If you get cramps during this exercise, your calcium is off. You can take a calcium/magnesium supplement for 1 month. If you get tired, your magnesium is out of balance. You can take a calcium/magnesium supplement for 1 month. If the arms hurt, your potassium is out of balance. You can eat 2 bananas, which have high potassium. If your lower back hurts, and you are a woman, menstruation is impaired. Eat more soy products, which contain isoflavones. If your lower back hurts, and you are a man, you may be on the verge of urological problems. In this case you should see a urologist. If your head hurts, it means the flow of blood to your head is obstructed and your nutrition is not right.

Part 2: This exercise brings the navel area into balance and recharges all the pranic areas and the immune system of the body. It will put you into a deep meditative state, even if done only for a few minutes.

MEDICAL MEDITATION FOR EPILEPSY

Tune in and center yourself by chanting "Ong Namo, Guru Dev Namo" 3 times (Tune on page 143).

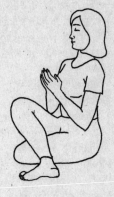

Posture: Sit on your left heel, right leg over the left, left leg touching the floor. This is called Hero Pose. You can also sit in a chair with your right leg crossed over your left knee and your back straight.

Focus: The eyes are one-tenth open and look at the palms of your hands.

Breath: The breath will come automatically as you chant.

Mantra: Chant continuously the mantra "Sa, Ta, Na, Ma."

Meaning of mantra: This mantra represents the cycle of creation. *Sa* means infinity; *Ta* means life; *Na* means death; *Ma* means rebirth.

Mudra: The hands are cupped, little fingers touching along their length, in front of your chest, as if you were about to receive an offering.

Time: Start with 3 or 11 minutes, and slowly build up to 31 minutes.

End: Inhale, hold your breath for 10 seconds, exhale, and relax.

COMMENTS: This Medical Meditation is helpful in cases of epilepsy. Of course, however, no patient should stop taking any antiseizure medication abruptly, or without the knowledge of his or her physician.

MEDICAL MEDITATION FOR MENTAL FATIGUE

Tune in and center yourself by chanting "Ong Namo, Guru Dev Namo" 3 times (Tune on page 143).

Posture: Sit in Easy Pose or in a chair with your spine straight.

Focus: The eyes are closed and focused at the third-eye point.

Breath: The breath will come automatically as you chant.

Mantra: Ong (pronounced "Ooonnnnnnnnnnnnnng"). This is chanted monotone, with your mouth open but the air flowing through your nose as you chant. The sound is far back and up in the soft palate.

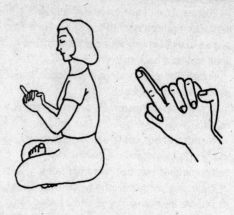

Meaning of mantra: *Ong* means Creator—the primal vibration from which all creativity flows.

Mudra: Place your ring fingers together and interlace all the other fingers, right thumb on top of the left. Hold your hands several inches out from your diaphragm with the ring fingers pointed upward at a 60 degree angle.

Time: 3 minutes.

End: Inhale deeply, hold your breath for 10–20 seconds, exhale, and relax.

COMMENTS: This Medical Meditation should only be done when you can relax afterward. Done correctly, it is very effective against brain drain. It also imparts a balanced mental state, and can give you absolutely powerful energy.

MEDICAL MEDITATION TO HELP PREVENT MIGRAINE HEADACHES

Tune in and center yourself by chanting "Ong Namo, Guru Dev Namo" 3 times (Tune on page 143).

Posture: Sit in Easy Pose or in a chair with your spine straight.

Focus: With your eyes closed, look at your hairline.

Breath: Long, slow, deep breathing.

Mantra: This Medical Meditation is done without a mantra.

Mudra: The hands are in gyan mudra, with the index fingers touching the thumbs. Extend the arms straight at a 70 degree angle out and up from the sides.

Time: 11 minutes.

End: Relax your hands onto the knees and chant, in a monotone, "We are the love," for 1–2 minutes. Then inhale deeply, hold your breath for 10 seconds, exhale, and relax.

COMMENTS: This Medical Meditation is indicated to help prevent migraines, especially if practiced over time. Avoid doing this during the headache. Pain in the back, and behind the shoulders, while doing this exercise, is a sign of weak blood circulation. If this happens, make sure you are getting regular aerobic exercise. A smoothie of bananas, soy milk, and a green drink powder will help. Besides helping with headaches, this meditation is great to release tension, tonify the liver, and open the lungs.

MEDICAL MEDITATION FOR DEPRESSION

Tune in and center yourself by chanting "Ong Namo, Guru Dev Namo" 3 times (Tune on page 143).

Posture: Sit in Easy Pose or in a chair with your spine straight.

Focus: Open your eyes and stare beyond your hands to the horizon. Keep your eyes fixed throughout the exercise. Meditate on the life energy of the breath.

Breath: Coordinate the breath with the movement and the mantra. All breathing is done through the nose.

Mantra: As your hands go out with the inhale, mentally vibrate "Sa"; as they return, mentally vibrate "Ta." For the second repetition, inhale and mentally vibrate "Na," exhale and mentally vibrate "Ma." The mental feeling of stretching your breath to a single point, to the width of your arms spread, is essential.

Meaning of mantra: This mantra represents the cycle of creation. *Sa* means infinity; *Ta* means life; *Na* means death; *Ma* means rebirth.

Mudra:

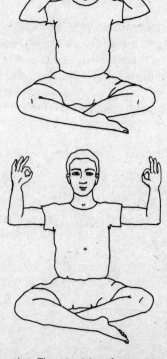

1. Start with your hands in gyan mudra, with the index finger touching your thumb. Bring the hands up in front of your eyes so that your thumbs and index fingers touch. The other fingers are straight and relaxed. Your upper arms are parallel to the floor.

2. Inhale and separate the hands outward 36 to 45 inches. Exhale and return to the original position. Your elbows will move a little, but keep them relaxed.

Time: Start with a slow movement, one cycle of the breath taking about 4 seconds. After 2 or 3 minutes increase the speed to 1 second per cycle, for a total of 4 seconds for each repetition of the mantra. Continue for 3 more minutes.

End: Inhale, exhale, and relax in Corpse Pose. Totally relax your arms and shoulders. Meditate at the crown chakra. If you must concentrate at all, focus all your energy at the top of the skull. Put all of your energy into total relaxation for 15 minutes.

COMMENTS: You are born to be positive and creative. The creativity of your existence is unlimited. Since we do not have the established habit of constancy in thought and action, we create negative patterns of thought, and depression. This Medical Meditation will let you evaluate and measure how positive or negative you are. It will also make you positive and happy. It focuses on the range of the breath. In the subconscious, breath and life are synonymous.

By meditating this way, depression can be alleviated. If you do it correctly, there will be a tremendous pressure at your lymph glands, located in your armpits.

MEDICAL MEDITATION FOR THE RELEASE OF SUBCONSCIOUS FEAR

Tune in and center yourself by chanting "Ong Namo, Guru Dev Namo" 3 times (Tune on page 143).

Posture: Sit in Easy Pose or in a chair with your spine straight.

Focus: The eyes are one-tenth open—the mental focus is at the third-eye point.

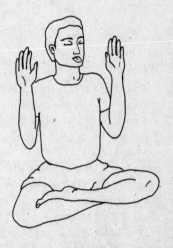

Breath: Extend your tongue out at its length. Lightly rest the top teeth across the tongue. Inhale through the mouth in a long, gentle breath, so that you can feel the breath along the sides of your tongue.

Mantra: On the inhalation, mentally repeat the sound "Go." Exhale through your nose, and mentally repeat the sound "Bind" (the sound "in" is pronounced like the word *in*). Here it is broken into two parts. *Go* is the sustaining factor that surrounds the essence, and *Bind* is the essence, the nucleus, the seed of the self; the inner point or center.

Meaning of mantra: The mantra "Gobind" is to sustain and protect the self.

Mudra: Bend your elbows so each hand is at ear level, just in front of you. Your palms are facing forward, flat open with your fingers pointing up. Elbows and arms are relaxed, and resting close to the body.

Time: 3–11 minutes.

End: Inhale deeply, bring your tongue back into your mouth, exhale, and stretch your hands and arms up.

COMMENTS: Sometimes at a very early age, fear becomes a part of our subconscious. As adults we may show this unconscious fear as fear of loss, separation, abandonment, or feelings of helplessness. Sometimes it shows itself in feelings of not really being sure of ourselves. This Medical Meditation will help release subconscious fear, and will give you a secure sense of yourself.

EASY MEDICAL MEDITATION FOR COGNITIVE FUNCTION

Tune in and center yourself by chanting "Ong Namo, Guru Dev Namo" 3 times (Tune on page 143).

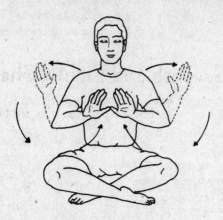

Posture: Sit in Easy Pose or in a chair with your spine straight.

Focus: The eyes are closed and focused at the third-eye point.

Breath: Breathing only through your nose, complete one breath per circle.

Mantra: This Medical Meditation is done without a mantra.

Mudra: Bend your elbows, keeping your hands at shoulder level, with your palms facing forward. Move your forearms in a fast, circular motion to the outside. As your hands pass the center of your chest, your thumbs touch slightly. Move as quickly as possible.

Time: 3–11 minutes.

End: Inhale at the starting position, hold your breath for 10 seconds, exhale. Repeat 2 more times.

COMMENTS: This Medical Meditation is helpful in improving coordination and focus.

CHAPTER SEVENTEEN

The Seventh and Eighth Chakras

Between Heaven and Earth

A Case History

HEALING WITH THE SEVENTH AND EIGHTH CHAKRAS

Lynn, a thirty-five-year-old woman, had symptoms of addiction to drugs. She was physically and psychologically dependent upon barbiturates. A well-known entertainment star, she had experimented with a wide range of drugs but had become addicted only to barbiturates. She had used heroin and cocaine sporadically, but did not appear to be addicted to either.

She had tried to overcome her addiction several times at various treatment centers, which had used a variety of approaches, including medication and counseling.

Then Lynn was placed on a program of Medical Meditation. She was not given medications, such as antidepressants, to help her taper off her drug use, as is conventional practice. Nor was she advised to undergo more counseling.

Her primary meditation was the Medical Meditation for Habituation or Addiction (see page 269). The vibratory effects from that meditation are particularly effective at stimulating the hypothalamic-pituitary-adrenocortical axis, or HPA axis. The HPA axis regulates endocrine secretions. I believed that this would help shift the entire profile of her endocrine secretions, neurotransmitter syntheses, and hormonal production. This approach was intended to enable her to replace her anxious, adrenergic psychophysical condition with a calm cholinergic healing condition.

This worked; it halted her overproduction of the adrenal hormone cortisol, which was extremely elevated, as it often is among substance abusers. It also increased her output of serotonin, which is generally in short supply among addicts. Often, cortisol and serotonin exist in the body in inverse proportions. When an imbalance favors cortisol, it greatly heightens vulnerability to many physical and emotional problems, including addiction. This imbalance often prompts addicts to self-medicate their innate biochemical disturbances.

Lynn's Medical Meditation also helped her psychologically. Her self-esteem increased, and she overcame a long-standing obsession with death, which had fueled her self-destructive impulses.

Today, Lynn is still drug-free after approximately five years.

The General Characteristics of the Seventh and Eighth Chakras

My patient's face was shadowed and haunted. There was an emptiness in his eyes that was as dark and hollow as the void of space. He was attending one of my Brain Longevity Seminars, in Tucson, because he'd begun to suffer from age-associated memory disorder. Increasingly, his mind was a thicket of confusion, pocked with black holes of lost memory.

At the end of that day's seminar, as the other attendees filed from the room, I pulled up a chair beside him, and we began to talk. He asked me some questions about the Medical Meditations for cognitive function that we had discussed that day. By way of answering his questions, I did a couple of meditations with him. He did them enthusiastically, and didn't miss a beat. When we finished, we both opened our eyes at the same time.

Even from that small effort, there seemed to be something new in his eyes—a connectedness, a spark. I relaxed my body and mind utterly, and focused all of my intuitive energy upon this sad, struggling man.

I picked up a strong feeling of what was going on inside him. After a moment, I said, "Know what I think? I think you're not here just to improve your memory. I think I know what the real problem is. I think that there's a deep spiritual longing in you." I repeated the phrase quietly: "A deep spiritual longing."

He looked shocked. And then his eyes glassed with tears. His words came out hesitantly, one at a time, from deep in the hollow of his belly. "I . . . think . . . you're . . . right." Then, more forcefully: "I think you're right!" His eyes were still wide with surprise, but then his gaze flipped suddenly inward. I sat with him, not speaking.

When he emerged from his introspection, several minutes later, it was as if I were looking at a person who had unexpectedly gotten a quick glimpse of a new selfhood. It wasn't his highest self that he'd seen—that could only come later, after a great deal more work. But it was his true self.

"You know," he said with a tone of conviction, but also amazement, "I think I've learned more about myself this afternoon than I learned in twenty years of psychotherapy!"

Truth be told, this brave man, with his pilgrim's soul, probably had not learned more on this afternoon than he had over the prior twenty years. But he had probably changed more. Learning is limited. Learning can awaken your head, but not your heart or your soul. Some of the most learned people I know are the least wise. They know too much and understand too little. Feeling, experiencing, doing—these are the acts that change our lives. These are the acts that pierce heart and soul. And these are the acts that Medical Meditation makes possible.

When this man traveled inside his own brain cells and memory synapses, via the vehicle of Medical Meditation, he met elements of himself that had long been hidden. He traveled beyond his rational self to his emotional self, and further still, to his spiritual self. That was the part of him he most needed to know. Without it, he could never be whole, and never be healed.

Remember, all healing begins with the mind—and the mind is the servant of the spirit. Spirituality cannot be attained just by thinking about it. To find it, you've got to feel it. Yet finding that feeling is impossible without the wondrous powers of the mind—the whole mind: the rational mind, the emotional mind, the intuitive mind, the mind that holds the past, the mind that conceives the future . . . and the mind that knows the soul.

Unfortunately, many people have little contact with the whole, united entirety of their minds. Instead, they are compartmentalized—separated in mind, body, and spirit—and this leaves them dull and dazed. They walk through life half-dead, experiencing little contact with the spirit that gives life to the mind, and the mind that gives life to the body. They just don't feel the united, whole energy that grants full being.

A fundamental reason for this common occurrence is weakness of the seventh and eighth chakras, the chakras that carry us to the realm of the spirit. All too often, though, people are so trapped in their lower, survival-oriented chakras that they fail to find the source of ultimate survival: the chakras of the spirit. Spirit is the only aspect of us that is truly immortal.

Your seventh chakra, or crown chakra, sits atop your head, near the area that was your soft spot when you were an infant. This chakra, along with the sixth chakra, governs the functions of the brain, and the pineal gland. Unlike the sixth chakra, though, it is only casually associated with the pituitary gland, which directs secretions to the body. Instead, the seventh chakra is far more focused on the universal, cosmic energy that enters the body, and exits the body, through the top of the head.

The seventh chakra is in overall, ultimate control of body, mind, and spirit, but can be activated only through the mind. When your crown chakra is open, you can actually merge with the energy of the cosmos and direct this energy toward your own healing. The crown chakra contains the human capacity for boundlessness. It is the spiritual center of the physical body.

The crown chakra is the pathway that allows us in and out of our bodies. It contains a strong sense of connection to our own personal vastness, as well as the vastness of the universe. It alone, of all the chakras, senses the creator within the creation, and the infinite within the finite. When this sensing occurs, you gain a feeling of security that is much greater than the personal security that emanates from the lower triangle of chakras (especially the solar plexus chakra). When your seventh chakra is open, you feel as if you are plugged into a power source that is completely dependable, and eternal.

The primary emotion that this connection causes is that of bliss. The blissful person lives neither in the heavens nor on the earth. This person instead brings heaven to earth, and earth to the heavens.

People who achieve the merging of heaven and earth, in their own lifetimes, have a unique, golden radiance, which transforms even their most mundane acts. For them, every effort is effortless. They are free. They are alive.

When life blooms full-flower within people, it energizes and enhances the final chakra: the eighth chakra, or aura. Interestingly, the eighth chakra—which is in some ways the most ethereal and mysterious chakra—is also the easiest chakra to locate and perceive in the material world. One reason for this is simply that the aura is external, and is therefore somewhat easier to identify physically. A number of scientific explorations have indicated the existence of the aura.

Virtually all anatomical researchers—even those who know nothing of auras—recognize the existence of a nonmaterial energy force that surrounds the body. The most simple, dross explanation for this energy field is that it is composed of the bioelectrical energy that exists in all living creatures.

You can feel this energy force yourself. Just open your hands, and place them facing each other, about an inch apart. Slowly move them slightly apart and slightly together, and focus on the feeling in your hands that this creates. Most people notice an energy force that feels somewhat like magnetic attraction and repulsion.

This energy force, though, can vary greatly in its intensity. Sometimes you can feel it with your hands several inches apart. Some people can even feel it with their hands up to twelve inches apart. The intensity of the force seems to wax and wane in relation to physical health, and spiritual strength. This variability, I believe, indicates that this force consists of much more than just standard human bioelectricity, which would not be expected to vary significantly over time, or during conditions of illness or health.

Furthermore, this energy has been captured on film, which would also be improbable if it were a bioelectric, or magnetic, force. For several decades now, researchers using the refined imaging technique of Kirlian photography have recorded images of the aura.

A number of highly attuned people appear to have the ability to see human auras, and this ability has been corroborated in clinical trials. For more than twenty years, neurophysiologist Valerie Hunt of UCLA has documented the ability of certain people to see auras. To do this, she had experienced aura readers note changes in the auras of volunteers, while she simultaneously monitored the volunteers with electronic methods, including electromyography. In virtually all of the trials she conducted, the changes perceived by the aura readers corresponded exactly to changes noted technologically. These changes included modifications of respiration rate, heart rate, blood pressure, and brain wave patterns.

Although the technological evidence of auras is of recent origin, people from diverse cultures have recorded perceptions of auras for many centuries. For example, many of the early religious paintings from the Middle Ages portrayed spiritual people with bright auras. In fact, many people believe that the concept of a halo is analogous to that of an aura. And even before the Middle Ages there were graphic depictions of auras in the art of the Egyptians and Persians.

Although most people cannot see auras, people who can see them believe that the majority of people could be trained to see them. There are various techniques that can help you to learn this skill, such as looking at yourself in a mirror without focusing your eyes directly upon your image.

Even people who cannot see auras can sometimes notice it when their own aura is visually pierced by another person. This occurs in the common situation in which a person suddenly feels as if she is being stared at, and then turns around and does, indeed, see someone staring at her. This interesting phenomenon has been tested technologically. Researchers using galvanic skin response monitors have noted changes in skin response that occurred the moment before a subject realized that he or she was being stared at.

Auras sometimes become weak and thin, if a person is sick, exhausted, or very spiritually depleted. However, in some vital and spiritual people, auras can extend for several feet. When people are quite ill, their auras can even collapse inward, and become virtually invisible. Some spiritual healers believe that when this occurs, it is wise to allow the aura to remain internal, because it is closely protecting the vital organs that must be nurtured to regain health. This inward refocus of the aura is similar to the drawing in of blood that occurs when a person is ill. Illness prompts the body to redirect blood flow to the internal organs, away from the skin and the extremities. This accounts for the common condition of being pale and having cold hands and feet when illness occurs.

Aura is derived from the Greek word for air, because the aura is in intimate, direct contact with the airlike ether, or ethereal energy, that permeates the universe. In the ancient Indian culture, the aura was thought to be directly connected to prana, and in the ancient Chinese culture, it was thought to be directly connected to *chi*.

In the kundalini yoga tradition, which is derived from the Indian culture, the aura is thought to be a highly effective shield against negative external forces. Therefore, if the aura is weak, it increases vulnerability to disease. Unfortunately, though, disease itself weakens the aura. Therefore, a negative spiral can occur, which can also affect the chakras, which are very closely connected to the aura. The aura is somewhat like a circumventive field, or filter, that shields and encloses the other seven chakras.

An important part of this protective field is the arc line, which is the segment of the aura that is our definitive early warning system. Those first danger signals that you sense when you are beginning to get sick are, I believe, not just symptoms of biochemical imbalance, but also perceptions of distress emanating from the arc line.

Among the most magical features of the aura is its ability to heal not only the person it belongs to, but also others. The ability of one individual to help heal another with his own aura has been well documented for some time. Touch healing is still considered controversial by staunchly orthodox physicians, but it is gradually entering the mainstream, as documentation of its validity continues to accumulate.

One reason that touch healing works is because the energies of your aura, unlike the energies of your lower chakras, do not consist solely of yourself. Instead, these energies consist of you plus the energies of the universe. These energies are not yours to have and to hold. They come and they go, like the wind, which is also invisible but still tangible. These energies are the sharing of you with others, the sharing of you with the universe, and the sharing of you with the divine spirit. These energies embody an eternal truth: all things come from God, and all things go to God.

The Physical Characteristics of the Seventh and Eighth Chakras

The eighth chakra, or aura, is far less involved with specific, discrete areas of the body. Much more than any other chakra, it is involved with the entire physical organism, as a whole.

The primary physical structure governed by the seventh chakra is the cerebrum, the upper part of the brain that performs cognitive functions. Most of the rest of the brain, including the brain stem and the cerebellum, governs physical actions and automatic instincts, and is governed by the sixth chakra.

The eighth chakra allows you to send positive healing energy to other people and is your projection to others that allows them to feel your presence. An expansive aura is a byproduct of Medical Meditation for this chakra.

The cerebrum weighs about two pounds, and is shaped somewhat like two halves of a walnut, joined together to form a sphere. It is covered by a layer of gray matter that is only about one to two millimeters thick. This gray matter composes the neocortex, and performs virtually all of the higher thought processes.

The cerebrum is divided into four lobes: (1) the frontal lobe, which solves abstract problems; (2) the parietal lobe, which sorts out messages from the senses; (3) the temporal lobe, which governs language, hearing, and memory; and (4) the occipital lobe, which controls vision.

It was once believed that particular types of memory—such as memories about family, or memories about work—were stored in localized compartments. It's now known, though, that memories exist as widely scattered networks of neuronal connections. Therefore, to function properly, the brain must have an abundance of the chemical neurotransmitters that connect one brain cell to another, and thus allow complex patterns of memories to exist.

Medical Meditation is particularly adept at helping to manufacture the neurotransmitters the brain needs. Each neurotransmitter is synthesized within the body from particular nutrients, and the physical exercises and pranayama breathing exercises of Medical Meditation enhance this synthesis by providing increased blood flow and increased oxygenation.

Medical Meditation also has notably salubrious effects upon the only endocrine gland directly governed by the seventh chakra, the pineal gland. The pineal gland was once believed to invariably wither and calcify during old age, but this belief has been challenged by practitioners of Medical Meditation and kundalini yoga. These people, who are able to back up their beliefs with evidence from advanced imaging techniques, think that specific exercises that heighten blood flow and energy flow to the pineal can prevent this common calcification.

When calcification does occur, it prohibits the production of the pineal hormone melatonin, which is best known as the sleep hormone. It's widely believed that this decline of melatonin creates the difficulty in achieving enough sleep that many older people experience. Besides helping initiate sleep, melatonin exerts a wide range of other activities, including boosting immunity. It's also a general feel-good hormone, the nighttime equivalent of serotonin.

Many people take melatonin supplements to compensate for the age-associated deterioration of the pineal, but I much prefer to mediate against this deterioration with Medical Meditation. I prefer Medical Meditation because it marshals the body's own natural powers, and because melatonin supplementation may someday be shown to have negative side effects.

As you probably know, the brain has two hemispheres that can function somewhat independently. However, optimal cognitive function occurs only when the two hemispheres are communicating with maximum efficiency. This communication occurs primarily via the band of nerve fibers that connects the two hemispheres, the corpus callosum. Women tend to have thicker, stronger corpus callosums than do men, and this creates some of the cognitive differences that appear to exist among males and females. One such difference is a higher incidence among men of problems such as dyslexia and hyperactivity, which are exacerbated by lack of hemispheric coordination. Another difference is a relatively heightened sense of intuition among women, due to their increased whole-brain communication.

Medical Meditation is an excellent modality for increasing hemispheric communication. It does this by bringing physical and ethereal energy to all parts of the brain, including the corpus callosum.

The elevated intuition that is created by Medical Meditation can be used to serve a lofty purpose. It can heighten the receptivity of the brain to perceptions that go unnoticed by the parts of the brain that process only logic. Chief among these are spiritual perceptions. The brain, at its highest level of function, is the antenna that receives the messages of the cosmos. These messages, often as not, are indescribably subtle. They may be nothing more than vibrations.

But these vibrations can be deciphered, and made sensible, if one's brain is empowered by intuition and vitality. With heightened attunement, a person can find words in these vibrations. The words can be a message from one's own heart. The words can be a message from a loved one, far away, long gone, never forgotten. Or the words can be the word of God. This is the blessing of the seventh chakra.

Medical Meditations for the Seventh and Eighth Chakras

SPECIAL MEDITATION FOR THE SEVENTH AND EIGHTH CHAKRAS

Tune in and center yourself by chanting "Ong Namo, Guru Dev Namo" 3 times (Tune on page 143).

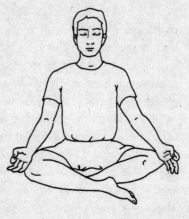

Posture: Sit in Easy Pose or in a chair with your spine straight.

Focus: The eyes are focused on the tip of the nose.

Breath: The breath will come automatically as you chant.

Mantra: "Ang Sang Wahe Guru."

Meaning of mantra: "God is in every cell of my body."

Mudra: The hands are in gyan mudra, with the index fingers touching the thumbs.

Time: 31 minutes.

End: Inhale deeply and hold your breath as long as possible. Exhale. Repeat 2 more times.

COMMENTS: This Medical Meditation will help you feel the beauty, bounty, and bliss of your own soul.

MEDICAL MEDITATION FOR HABITUATION OR ADDICTION

Tune in and center yourself by chanting "Ong Namo, Guru Dev Namo" 3 times (Tune on page 143).

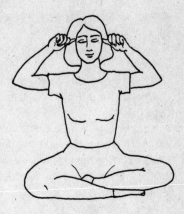

Posture: Sit in Easy Pose or in a chair with your spine straight. Make sure that your lowest 6 vertebrae are pushed forward.

Focus: The eyes are closed and focused at the third-eye point.

Breath: The breath will come automatically as you chant.

Mantra: "Sa, Ta, Na, Ma." Lock your back molars and keep your lips closed. Vibrate your jaw muscles by alternating the pressure on your molars.

Meaning of mantra: This mantra represents the cycle of creation. *Sa* means infinity; *Ta* means life; *Na* means death; *Ma* means rebirth.

Mudra: Make fists of your hands. Extend your thumbs straight and place them on your temples in the niche where they fit.

Time: 5–7 minutes to start. With practice you can build up to 20–31 minutes.

End: Inhale deeply, hold your breath for 10–20 seconds, exhale and relax.

COMMENTS: The yogis say that this Medical Meditation is one of a class of meditations that will become well-known to the future medical society.

The pressure exerted by the thumbs triggers a rhythmic reflex current into the central brain. This current activates the brain area directly underneath the stem of the pineal gland. It is said that it is an imbalance in this area that makes mental and physical addictions seemingly unbreakable.

In modern culture, the imbalance is pandemic. If we are not addicted to smoking, eating, drinking, or drugs, then we are addicted subconsciously to acceptance, advancement, rejection, emotional love, etc. All these lead us to insecure and neurotic behavior patterns.

The imbalance in this pineal area upsets the radiance of the pineal gland itself. It is this pulsating radiance that regulates the pituitary gland. Since the pituitary regulates the rest of the glandular system, the entire body and mind go out of balance. This Medical Meditation helps to correct this problem. It is excellent for everyone but particularly effective for rehabilitation efforts in drug dependence, mental illness, and phobic conditions.

MEDICAL MEDITATION TO OPEN THE CROWN CHAKRA

Tune in and center yourself by chanting "Ong Namo, Guru Dev Namo" 3 times (Tune on page 143).

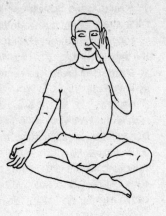

1. Posture: Sit in Easy Pose or in a chair with your spine straight.

Focus: With the eyes closed, focus at the third-eye point.

Breath: Breath of Fire through the right nostril.

Mantra: This Medical Meditation is done without a mantra.

Mudra: Block your left nostril with the thumb of your left hand, with the fingers pointing straight up. The right hand is relaxed on your right knee in gyan mudra, with the index finger touching the thumb.

Time: 3 minutes.

End: Inhale deeply, hold, and savor the breath for 10 seconds; exhale, relax, and meditate for 3 minutes.

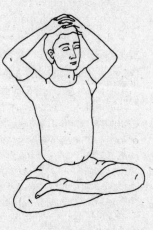

2. Posture: Sit in Easy Pose or in a chair with your spine straight.

Focus: With the eyes closed, focus on your crown chakra. Press your tongue on the roof of your mouth.

Breath: Breath of Fire.

Mantra: This Medical Meditation is done without a mantra.

Mudra: Put your hands in Venus lock (see page 96 for reference) and place them above the top of your head (directly over the crown chakra).

Time: 3 minutes.

End: Inhale deeply, hold the breath for 10 seconds, then exhale. Repeat 2 more times, then relax.

COMMENTS: This Medical Meditation helps bring energy and balance to the seventh chakra, or crown chakra, the part of your ethereal being that is most closely attuned to the energies of the universe.

This is a very simple yet effective Medical Meditation. If you are a beginner, you may start by doing each part for 1 minute and gradually build up to the prescribed time.

MEDICAL MEDITATION TO TRANSFER HEALING ENERGY

Tune in and center yourself by chanting "Ong Namo, Guru Dev Namo" 3 times (Tune on page 143).

1. Posture: Sit in Easy Pose or in a chair with your spine straight.

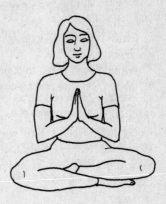

Focus: With the eyes closed, concentrate on the heart chakra. Let hate depart, fill the heart with love.

Breath: Long, slow, deep breathing through the nose.

Mantra: This Medical Meditation is done without a mantra.

Mudra: Bring your hands into prayer mudra, together at the center of your chest. Press your hands against each other with all the power you can muster.

Time: 4 minutes.

2. In the same position, now think of someone you love very much and send that person healing thoughts. Healing thoughts can be transmitted like radio waves; fill the whole room with them. Project them to the person you love.

End: Inhale deeply, fill your chest with love, and project pranic energy like a thunderbolt to the one you love. Exhale, inhale, and send the energy of this breath to the person on whom you are meditating. Exhale. Inhale again, and feel energy flowing from your hands to the person. Create a mental link. Feel the energy massaging the person. Exhale. Continue this energy massage for 1–3 minutes.

COMMENTS: This Medical Meditation is a direct healer. By combining the power of love with positive intention, and coloring it with prana, you can help someone heal.

MEDICAL MEDITATION TO HEAL SELF AND OTHERS

Tune in and center yourself by chanting "Ong Namo, Guru Dev Namo" 3 times (Tune on page 143).

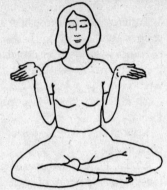

Posture: Sit in Easy Pose or in a chair with your back straight.

Focus: The eyes are nine-tenths closed.

Breath: The breath will come automatically as you chant. Inhale completely before you start chanting.

Mantra: "Ra Ma Da Sa, Sa Se So Hung." The mantra should be sung in one complete exhalation. As you chant the first "Sa," your navel point is pulled in so that this syllable is abbreviated. You should rest for 4 beats between the first "Sa" and the second "Sa."

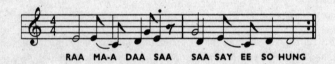

RAA   MA-A   DAA   SAA   SAA   SAY   EE   SO   HUNG

Meaning of mantra: This mantra literally means "I am Thou," but is also used to mean, "The service of God is within me."

Mudra: The hands are parallel with and facing the ceiling; fingers are together and pulled down. Your elbows are snug at your sides with the forearms in close to your upper arms. Your hands are at a 60-degree angle, halfway between pointing forward and pointing to the sides.

Time: 11 minutes. Very gradually, over a period of years, the time may be increased to a maximum of 31 minutes.

End: Inhale deeply, hold your breath, and visualize the person you want to send healing to. Make that image in your mind very clear and see a glowing green light around the person. Keeping that vision in your mind, exhale. Inhale deeply, hold your breath, and continue to send the person green healing light. Still keeping that vision in your mind, exhale. For the last time, inhale deeply, hold your breath and see the person very clearly, and see the green healing light bathing the person, bathing every cell in the body. Exhale and relax.

COMMENTS: Strive to maintain your chant at full volume (loud, but not raucous) throughout the meditation.

This highly effective meditation deals with *vayu siddhi*, the power of air. It brings health and many other desirable positive changes. If you wish to heal yourself, imagine a glowing green light around yourself as you meditate.

MEDICAL MEDITATION TO BRING LIGHT TO ALL THE CHAKRAS

I've saved the best for last. This is a great meditation. This Medical Meditation cuts through the darkness of neurotic thought. It helps to relieve the first chakra's unhealthy attachment to past traumas. It purifies your karma, and gives you the pranic power of health and healing. A recently published medical study showed it to be more effective than antidepressant medication in treating psychological issues.

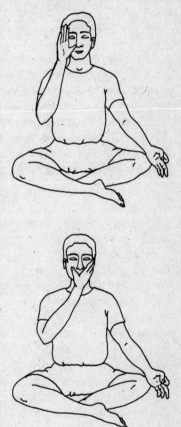

Tune in and center yourself by chanting "Ong Namo, Guru Dev Namo" 3 times (Tune on page 143).

Posture: Sit in Easy Pose or in a chair, with your spine straight and chin in.

Focus: The eyes are focused at the tip of your nose, or closed and focused at the third-eye point, as you prefer.

Breath: Block off your right nostril with your right thumb, all the other fingers are straight and pointed up. Breathe in through your left nostril, then relax your left hand on your left knee. As you hold your breath, mentally chant "Wha-Hey Guru" 16 times. Every time you repeat each word, pull in your navel point—once on *Wha,* once on *Hey,* and once for *Guru,* for all the 16 times of the repetition of the mantra (for a total of 48 pumps). Then block off your left nostril with your right index finger, and exhale slowly and deeply through your right nostril. Continue.

Mantra: "Wahe Guru."

Meaning of mantra: "Ecstasy of infinite consciousness, which brings me from darkness to light."

Mudra: The left hand is resting on the left knee in gyan mudra, with the index finger touching the thumb. The right hand is used to block off the nostrils, as described above.

Time: Suggested length of this Medical Meditation is 31–62 minutes a day. If you are a beginner, you can start with 3 minutes and gradually build up to 11 minutes and so on.

End: Inhale, hold your breath for 5–10 seconds, exhale. Then stretch up and shake every part of your body for about 1 minute, so that the energy may spread.

COMMENTS: This Medical Meditation is called Sodarshan Chakra Kriya.

> There is no time, no place, no space, and no condition attached to this mantra. Each garbage pit has its own time to clear. If you are going to clean your own garbage, you can clean it as fast as you can, or as slowly as you want.
>
> —*Yogi Bhajan*

11 minutes a day of this Medical Meditation can build your confidence and capacity to understand who you are; 31 minutes a day will give you great strength and discipline; 1 year will make you feel fantastic; 1,000 days of doing this Medical Meditation, and no one will be able to match your strength.

This Medical Meditation helps inner happiness, and ecstasy in life. It gives you a new start, against all odds. When external pressure becomes too great, it brings power from the inside. This Medical Meditation is said to be the most powerful kriya in the history of yoga. Now you have it as your own. Wahe Guru.

Epilogue

I once told Nicole, my patient who used Medical Meditation to help recuperate from a paralyzing injury, that all fear starts with the fear of death. As Nicole found out during her heroic battle against paralysis, only the spirit can carry us from the shadow of death, and free us from fear. And only then can we heal.

Usually young people—especially children—are free from the fear of death. They feel immortal. I've often wondered why. Is it because, for them, death, simply and obviously, is somewhat further away? Probably not. Most people just aren't that myopic, not even most children. I think the main reason they're free from this fear is even more simple, and more obvious: they don't fear death because they are so full of life.

The young are blessed. Life fills their spirit, and spirit fills their life. As we struggle to survive and succeed, though, loss and pain shatter the spirit, and dim its radiance. And so, too often, as the years pass by, we find ourselves wiser but weaker—oftentimes ill—faded in spirit, full of doubt, dark with fear. Death begins to stalk us, to overtake us.

But the spirit is immortal! It can be damaged but never destroyed. That is the divine gift to the mortal being. It is our link to divinity itself. The spirit, no matter how battered, can always be revived. This is the lesson the ancient masters taught. This is the lesson I have tried to pass on in this book.

The spirit can be summoned once more with the application of Medical Meditation. Medical meditation, unlike any other medical or philosophical approach, can spark the spirit, and unite the mutually supportive energies of the spirit, mind, and body. Once united, this sacred triad can exert otherworldly powers of healing.

When the beaten-down body and the mortal mind are ill and angry, frail and grieving, the spirit—no matter how dimmed by suffering—can still bring nurturance. And this nurturance, like the love of a mother for her baby, is always welcomed—and always returned.

Thus begins the cycle of healing. It isn't always easy. Medical Meditation is not an aspirin, which can be swallowed and forgotten. It is a process that is equal in power only to the energy of one's daily practice, or sadhana.

But this process, or path, can lead to more than the mere healing of disease. The path can lead to one's highest self. It can lead out of darkness, into light. It can lead to boundlessness—and even infinity. That is the blessing of illness. That is the blessing of healing. That is the blessing of life. May this blessing be bestowed upon you. *Sat Nam.*

Resources and Referrals

- To schedule a personalized Medical Meditation or Brain Longevity consultation with Dharma Singh Khalsa, M.D.;
- For a presentation on music, meditation, and healing by Dr. Dharma Singh Khalsa and his musical group, Bliss; and
- For tapes of each mantra with music, and CDs on Medical Meditation, please contact:

> Dharma Singh Khalsa, M.D.
> 2420 N. Pantano Road
> Tucson, AZ 85715
> Phone: (520) 749-8374
> Fax: (520) 296-6640
> e-mail: Drdharma @aol.com
> www.brain-longevity.com
> www.meditation-as-medicine.com

- If you are interested in seeing Dr. Khalsa's line of antiaging nutritional products for brain longevity, chronic pain, and Medical Meditation, please contact:

> Vitamin Research Products
> 3579 Highway 50 East
> Carson City, NV 89701
> Phone: (888) 234-0459
> www.brain-longevity.com
> www.meditation-as-medicine.com

- If you are interested in staying up to date on Dr. Khalsa's research on brain longevity and Medical Meditation, or if you would like to support the research of the nonprofit Alzheimer's Prevention Foundation, please contact:

The Alzheimer's Prevention Foundation
2420 N. Pantano Road
Tucson, AZ 85715
Phone: (520) 749-8374
Fax: (520) 296-6640
e-mail: AlzPrvFdn@aol.com
www.AlzheimersPrevention.org

- For a referral to a certified kundalini yoga teacher in your area, please contact:

  International Kundalini Yoga Teachers Association
  Route 2, Box 4, Shady Lane
  Española, NM 87532
  Phone: (505) 753-0423
  Fax: (505) 753-5982
  e-mail: ikyta@3ho.org
  www.yogibhajan.com

- To contact Cameron Stauth:

  Cameron Stauth
  e-mail: Stauth@teleport.com

Recommended Reading

Herbert Benson, M.D. *The Relaxation Response.* New York: William Morrow & Co., 1975. The all-time classic introductory book to basic meditation.

Yogi Bhajan, Ph.D. *The Master's Touch.* Los Angeles, Calif.: Kundalini Research Institute, 1997. A high-level discussion of advanced meditation.

———. *The Mind: Its Projections and Multiple Facets.* Los Angeles, Calif.: Kundalini Research Institute, 1998. An expansive discussion on developing the higher facets of your mind.

Deepak Chopra, M.D. *Quantum Healing: Exploring the Frontiers of Mind/Body Medical Meditation.* New York: Bantam Books, 1989. A seminal discussion of the profound effects of meditation.

Dharma Singh Khalsa, M.D., with Cameron Stauth. *Brain Longevity: The Breakthrough Medical Program That Improves Your Mind and Memory.* New York: Warner Books, 1997. Introduces the concept of medical meditation and presents mind-body exercises specific for enhancing cognitive power.

———. *The Pain Cure: The Proven Medical Program That Helps End Your Chronic Pain.* New York: Warner Books, 1999. Expands Dr. Khalsa's work on specific meditation techniques for different ailments.

Gurucharan Singh Khalsa, Ph.D. *Breathwalk.* New York: Broadway Books, 2000. Describes how to breathe and meditate for an enhanced walking experience.

Shakti Parwha Kaur Khalsa. *Kundalini: The Flow of Power.* New York: Berkeley/Penguin Putnam, 1998. An excellent introductory book on kundalini yoga.

Sadhana Guidelines. Los Angeles, Calif.: Kundalini Research Institute, 1985. Many examples of yoga sets and meditations to begin your day.

Regarding Scientific References

Literally thousands of articles are available regarding academic research on mind-body interactions, Transcendental Meditation, mindfulness meditation, the relaxation response, and Medical Meditation.

As this book is for the general reading public, I have chosen not to include them. If, however, a scientific research bibliography is of interest to you, I will be pleased to mail one to you. The best way is to e-mail me with your mailing address, and one will be sent out.

Thank you in advance for understanding my humble attempt to save a few trees and heal the planet.

Blessings,

Dharma Singh Khalsa, M.D.

Acknowledgments

First and foremost, I must thank my teacher, His Holiness Siri Singh Sahib Yogi Bhajan, Ph.D., master of kundalini and white tantric yoga. May I also humbly bow before the golden chain of teachers, including Sant Hazara Singh, and, of course, Guru Ram Das, known as the Fourth Master, who lived in sixteenth-century India. I also make supplication before the Siri Guru Granth Sahib.

Deepest appreciation to Bhai Avtar Singh Ragi, Bhai Swaran Singh Ragi, Bhai Tej Pal Singh Ragi, and Bhai Baldeep Singh Ragi for the power of their prayers and the blessing of the naad.

Great gratitude to Judith Curr, president, publisher, and editor-in-chief of Pocket Books, for her clear, strategic vision of our work. Tracy Behar, our personal editor at Pocket Books, shared her talent, friendship, support, and guidance. She is a clear light, and I am very grateful to her. Also, thanks to Brenda Copeland, Tracy's assistant, and everyone else at Pocket Books for their help.

Cam Stauth, a professional's professional, made this book happen. Cam never ceases to amaze me with his dedication and skill. Thanks also to Sandra Stahl, our transcriptionist, whose work was superb and above and beyond the call of duty. I am also very grateful to Joan Borysenko, Ph.D., for her friendship and support, and for writing the foreword.

I could not have proceeded without the research help and shared knowledge of the following fellow students of Yogi Bhajan: Gurucharan Singh Khalsa, Ph.D., Shanti Shanti Kaur Khalsa, Ph.D., Shakti Parwha Kaur Khalsa, Livtar Singh Khalsa, Guru Singh Khalsa, Guru Tej Singh Khalsa, and Sadhana Kaur Khalsa, M.D. Thanks to Siri Kartar Kaur Khalsa, Guru Parkash Singh Khalsa, and Guru Fateh Singh Khalsa for the illustrations.

Carol Khalsa, the executive director of the Alzheimer's Prevention Foundation, has worked hard to bring our work to the attention of the academic community and the lay public. She and her husband, Darshan Singh Khalsa, are great supporters and friends. Thanks also to Mrs. Alma Robson, Mrs. Nell Singer, Ron

Lawrence, Ph.D., M.D., Dr. Ron Klatz, president of the American Academy of Anti-Aging Medicine, and the estate of Marjorie Olmstead.

Others who have been supportive of my work include Deepak Chopra, M.D.; Arielle Ford; Elisabeth Targ, M.D.; Larry Dossey, M.D.; Lyle Hurd, publisher of *Total Health* magazine; Hal Zina Bennett, Ph.D.; Kyle Roderick; Ruth Buczynski, Ph.D., of the National Institute for the Clinical Application of Behavioral Medicine; Joseph DeNucci, general manager, and Nordine Zouareg, M.A., director, of the Body Mindfulness Center; and Madeleine Randall, M.D., medical director, Miraval Life in Balance Resort; and Rob Watson, president and CEO of Vitamin Research Products. Also, Somers White, CPAE, CSP, the top guru, as a management consultant and coach. Somers has performed thirty assignments for me, all with superb results. Dick Onsager, my attorney, is always there for us with great advice and expertise.

Finally, please let me thank my agent, Richard Pine, who as usual had the clarity, vision, and capacity to bring this important work to you. Three down, and many more to go.

All of us, working together, have applied a great deal of positive healing energy, intention, projection and purpose to make *Meditation as Medicine* available to activate your natural healing force.

All love and blessings,

Dharma Singh Khalsa, M.D.
Tucson, Arizona

I would like to thank Richard Pine, my agent for twenty-five years, for having the creative vision that inspired this book. Thanks also to Korri Irvin, who helped me with the initial research. I'm also grateful to Sandra Stahl, who helped complete the book, and worked always with an ethic of professionalism and excellence.

Cameron Stauth
Portland, Oregon

Index

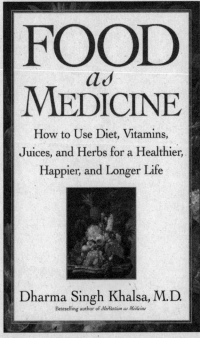